Sarah Clement is a resea... psychology degree, and v... University of London, wri... traditionally male jobs. She is herself a caesarean mother and helps to run one of the National Childbirth Trust's caesarean support groups. She is married and has two sons, Joel and Calum.

THE
CAESAREAN
EXPERIENCE

SARAH
CLEMENT

Pandora
An Imprint of HarperCollins Publishers

For Joel

Pandora Press
An Imprint of HarperCollins*Publishers*
77 — 85 Fulham Palace Road
London, W6 8JB

Published by Pandora Press 1991
1   3   5   7   9   10   8   6   4   2

A catalogue record for this book
is available from the British Library

ISBN 0 04 440738 6

Typeset by Harper Phototypesetters Limited,
Northampton, England
Printed in Great Britain by
HarperCollinsManufacturing Glasgow

Contents

Acknowledgements   7

Foreword by Sheila Kitzinger   8

Introduction   13

1 Why a Caesarean?   17

Disproportion, 18; Failure to Progress, 19; Fetal Distress, 21; Breech Baby, 23; Transverse Lie, 25; Malposition, 25; Previous Caesarean, 26; Placenta Praevia, 28; Antepartum Haemorrhage, 28; Prolapsed Cord, 29; Vulnerable Babies, 30; Problems in the Mother, 31; The Rising Caesarean Birth Rate, 32; Non-medical Factors, 35.

2 The Easy Way to Have a Baby?   40

A Pain-free Delivery?, 41; Great Expectations, 41; A Healthy Mother and Baby Are All That Matters?, 43; It's All in the Hands of the Doctors?, 44; You'll Feel Like Any Other Mother?, 45; A Risk-free Delivery?, 46.

3 Born a Cut Above   49

An Emergency or an Elective Caesarean, 49; The Anaesthetic Decision, 52; What Happens, 56; How it Feels, 60; Anaesthetic Failure, 65; Perceptions of Necessity, 68; The Importance of Being Involved and Informed, 69; Care and Support During Childbirth, 72.

4 Early Days   74

The Hospital Stay, 74; Coping with Pain, 78; Caring for Your Baby, 80; On an Emotional Rollercoaster, 82; Coming Home, 84; Physical Recovery, 88; The First Steps to Emotional Recovery, 91.

5 The Wound in the Mind   93

A Loss to be Mourned, 96; Altered Identities, 100; Intimations of Mortality, 102; Violation, 104; A Sense of Betrayal, 105; Post-traumatic Stress, 107; Postnatal Depression, 107.

6 Mother and Child   111
Bonds of Love, 111; Babies in Special Care, 114; When a Baby Dies, 117; Breastfeeding After a Caesarean, 118; Maternal Perceptions, 124; A Child's-eye View, 127.

7 Partners' Perspectives   133
A Father's Place, 133; Being There, 139; Pacing the Corridor, 140; Father and Child, 142; Mixed Emotions, 143; Your Relationship After a Caesarean, 146.

8 Coming to Terms   149
Talking It Through, 151; Missing Pieces, 155; Cause for Complaint, 158; Focusing on the Positive, 160; A New Perspective, 161.

9 Next Time   164
Another Baby?, 164; Another Caesarean?, 167; Trials and Tribulations, 178; Scar Separation in Perspective, 178; Degrees of Intervention, 180; Home Birth, 187; Caesarean Birth Second Time Around, 188; The VBAC Experience, 193.

10 What is to be Done   195
Caesarean Prevention, 195; Helping Yourself to a Better Caesarean, 201; Every Caesarean a Good Caesarean, 204.

Notes   211
Glossary of Terms   227
Further Reading   233
Useful Addresses   235
Index   237

ACKNOWLEDGEMENTS

First and foremost I would like to thank all those women who shared their experiences of caesarean childbirth with me. Their accounts have enriched and deepened my understanding of caesarean birth, and its meaning to women who give birth this way. Their words are reproduced throughout this book to speak of and document the caesarean experience. I would also like to thank the Caesarean Support Network, the National Childbirth Trust and *Practical Parenting* magazine for helping to put me in contact with these women.

A number of people have made suggestions and helpful comments on earlier drafts of this book, although the responsibility for the final manuscript rests with me. I would like to thank Candida Lacey and Ginny Iliff at Pandora Press; Midwives Rebecca Reed and Lucyann Davies; and friends and fellow caesarean mothers, Teresa Hamlin and Christina Viti. Their feedback and enthusiasm were much appreciated.

I would also like to thank my father, Bob Clement, who drew the illustrations. In addition, I would like to acknowledge those authors upon whose work I have drawn quite extensively, that is Murray Enkin, Marc J.N.C. Keirse and Iain Chalmers, *A Guide to Effective Care in Pregnancy and Childbirth*, Oxford University Press, Oxford, 1989; and Nancy Wainer Cohen and Lois J. Estner, *Silent Knife: Cesarean Prevention and Vaginal Birth after Cesarean*, Bergin and Garvey, Massachusetts, 1983; and those I have quoted at length, namely April Altman, 'From ICU to Empirical Midwifery' in Lynn Baptisti Richard's book *The Vaginal Birth After Cesarean Experience: Birth Stories by Parents and Professionals*, Bergin and Garvey, Massachusetts, 1987.

Most importantly, I would like to thank my husband, Steve Bowen, for his continuing emotional support and encouragement, for his unstinting belief in the importance of this book, for his suggestions and comments on earlier drafts, and for his practical help in assisting with the statistical analysis and in checking the text for errors and inconsistencies.

Lastly, I would like to thank my son, Joel, whose birth gave me the inspiration to write this book.

Foreword

by
SHEILA KITZINGER

It is a shock to learn that you must have a caesarean section, and one that is more difficult to handle if the decision is made during labour rather than if surgery is planned in advance. For emotional adjustment to the idea of caesarean section takes time.

After a caesarean, too, however happy you are to have your baby at last, you may wonder if it was really necessary, and if you could have avoided it by taking some positive action. Many women feel a sense of guilt, inadequacy and even stigma. In my experience, listening to women talk about how they are trying to cope with their mixed feelings after childbirth, there is usually a delay of some months before these negative emotions flood in, and then some women become overwhelmed with distress. At first a new mother is enormously grateful that she has a live, healthy baby, but later, as she reflects on the birth, she may come to feel that she was treated simply as a container for the fetus, that she was not given the chance to labour normally because so many interventions took place, and that she had no real choices. This makes her angry with the professionals who managed her labour. But because they have been kind and supportive, she believes that she really has no 'right' to express that anger, and she represses it. So it is turned in onto herself, and becomes depression. She is experiencing these powerful emotions at a time when other people consider that she should 'be over it by now' and that she should 'pull herself together'.[1]

On the other hand, a woman may feel that caesarean section is a wonderful way to have a baby, and hope that she can have a caesarean next time, too. Vaginal birth may seem quite frightening compared with a well-managed caesarean birth when the mother is kept fully informed and feels that she is in good hands.

Even with the first baby, some women prefer the idea of a

caesarean rather than a vaginal birth. They may believe that a caesarean section offers the solution to pain, without understanding that there is always post-operative pain, and hope that it will save them from what they see as the whole messy business of vaginal birth. Some even believe that a caesarean has advantages because they keep their passages 'honeymoon fresh' and that it is less physically damaging than vaginal birth because all they would be left with is a tiny scar that can be hidden under a bikini. There are women, too, who think that it is a more 'human' and less 'animal' way of having a baby. Many believe that, above all, it is safer for the baby. They have been misled. Yes, of course, when there is *placenta praevia* (that is when the placenta is practically or completely over the cervix), caesarean section is safer than vaginal birth, and there are some other situations in which it is difficult for a baby to be born vaginally. But, in general, caesarean section is not safer for the baby.

One in every 8 or 9 mothers in Britain, and one in every 4 in the USA, give birth by caesarean section. In some parts of the USA, every second woman can expect a caesarean birth. For there is today what amounts to an epidemic of caesarean sections in the western world, an epidemic that is fast spreading to the developing countries. How has this happened?

One reason is the rapid, wholesale introduction of electronic fetal monitoring, without adequate research and supported by an indiscriminating faith in technology. The use of the electronic fetal monitor accounts for approximately one-third of the increase in caesarean sections.[2] An electronic fetal monitor records many variations in the fetal heart rate that still come as a surprise to caregivers because normal variations — when the baby is sleeping, for example — are often not fully understood. Moreover, the machinery may produce variations which are artefacts of the technology itself, rather than an accurate record of the fetal heart rate. The result is that obstetricians become anxious and tend to opt for emergency caesarean sections.

When a woman has already had one caesarean, many American obstetricians believe that her other births should also be caesareans, and repeat operations account for over 30 per cent of caesarean births. Fortunately, this has never been the case in Britain, where most doctors expect a normal birth unless the same condition that resulted in the previous caesaerean recurs. Even so, British obstetricians are generally only happy for a woman to have a trial of labour if she will accept high levels of intervention.

In the USA, litigation against obstetricians who have failed to produce a perfect baby also pushes doctors into doing caesareans. Increasingly, obstetricians in Europe, too, say that they feel under pressure to intervene 'just in case' they might be accused of negligence later.

Everywhere private patients have more caesarean sections than those in any national health service. In Brazil, around 75 per cent of private patients are delivered by caesarean, compared with 25 per cent of clinic patients. The most privileged women are the least privileged when it comes to having the opportunity to go for spontaneous vaginal birth.

There is no evidence that high caesarean section rates are saving babies' lives, or producing healthier babies. There is evidence that caesarean section increases the risk of birth to mothers, and that it leads to more illness afterwards, especially from infection. So it is women who are paying the price for these high caesarean rates.

Caesarean section is a major operation, one that is simple for doctors to perform, and that can be done in only a few minutes (with the stitching up afterwards taking far longer). But it is usually followed by acute pain for which a woman requires drugs for pain relief, and she needs time to recover from the operation, as after any other surgery. This might be easy to organise, except that now she is coping with a new baby, and experiencing the important life transition that the birth of the baby brings with it.

Caesarean birth is for many women not only physically but also emotionally traumatic. As one woman told me, 'Pregnancy and birth are a bit like the build-up to Christmas. Suddenly it is all taken away from you and a momentous event you prepared yourself for is out of your control.'

The resulting emotional challenge is not just a matter of disappointment and feeling 'let down'. An unexpected caesarean may be experienced as a violent assault, however kindly the care is given, and even though a woman accepts that it was urgently necessary to save her baby. In fact, however, when caesarean section is performed for fetal distress, it is often discovered at delivery that the baby is perfectly all right. Everyone is delighted about this, of course, but later it may dawn on the woman that she has had an unnecessary caesarean.

Anyone who had looked forward to a birth in which she can be active and who wants as little interference as possible, is likely to feel cheated when she has a caesarean section. She may even feel a failure as a woman and guilty that she is herself responsible for things going wrong. It does not help when other people tell her to count her blessings and to be grateful that she has a healthy baby, or when they imply that she has somehow got off lightly because she did not have to deliver the baby herself. A woman who was expecting an elective (planned in advance) caesarean told me that a friend phoned to say, 'Lucky you! You've chosen the soft option, I see!'

Many women who have had a caesarean are determined to do everything they can in a subsequent pregnancy to avoid a repeat caesarean. So they ask for a VBAC — Vaginal Birth After Caesarean. In the USA, the Department of Health and Human Services, after lengthy investigations, declared VBAC to be low risk as long ago as 1981. This was followed by similar statements from the American College of Obstetrics and Gynecology, and the Society of Obstetricians and Gynecologists of Canada the year after. Yet there are still obstetricians who refuse to let women have a 'trial of labour', and some are not above employing emotional blackmail, telling the woman that she will be responsible for killing her baby or causing brain damage. In the United States and Canada, 9 out of every 10 women undergo a repeat caesarean section.

The major reason why obstetricians refuse to do a VBAC is that they are anxious that the wall of the weakened uterus will rupture. Canadian research into close on 53,000 of all births that took place in a particular hospital over a twenty-year period reveals that the risk of this occurring is of the order of 0.3 per cent per thousand births; that in half the cases where rupture occurs the woman has not had a previous caesarean birth; and that even in the few cases when a scar unpeels, not a single mother and not a single baby died as a result.[3]

Birth tends to be more difficult for a baby who is born bottom first — a breech — because the head is the largest part and the body may slip through before the birth passage is wide enough open to enable the head to slide out easily. There are obstetricians who believe it is right to section all women with breech babies, perhaps because they are not confident of their clinical skills in delivering a breech vaginally. Yet there is no reliable research to suggest that delivering all these babies by caesarean section will save lives.

It is important for any woman who might be told that she needs a caesarean section to be aware of these findings, so that she knows the right questions to ask, can share in decision-making and, when necessary, can challenge medical authoritarianism.

Sarah Clement, who has personal experience of both caesarean and vaginal birth, writes about these issues on the basis of her own in-depth psychological research. With clarity and with keen understanding, she explores ways of meeting the challenge of this different kind of birth.

Sheila Kitzinger

[1] Sheila Kitzinger, 'Birth and violence against women' in Helen Roberts (ed.), *Women's Health Matters*, London, Routledge, 1991.
[2] A. Grant, 'Monitoring the fetus during labour' in Iain Chalmers, Murray Enkin and Marc J.N.C. Keirse (eds), *Effective Care In Pregnancy And Childbirth*, Oxford, Oxford University Press, 1989.
[3] D.M. Fedorkow, C.A. Nimrod, P.J. Taylor, 'Ruptured uterus in pregnancy: a Canadian hospital's experience' in *Canadian Medical Association Journal*, no. 137, 1987, pp. 27-9.

Introduction

We are the growing and forgotten band of childbearers.

Caesarean childbirth is a major life experience. When we give birth by caesarean we undergo major abdominal surgery, often in an emergency situation or at short notice; we begin a new relationship of central importance in our lives, that is the relationship with our newborn baby; and we start the new and demanding job of caring for our infants — all at the same time! As such we may experience caesarean birth as either an emotional and bodily challenge from which we may grow and feel strengthened, having met the challenge. It may equally be experienced as an overwhelming psychological and physical crisis which leaves us feeling profoundly distressed and deeply wounded.

This book is about how it feels to have a baby by caesarean. In the three years since the caesarean birth of my son, I read everything I could find on caesarean childbirth, and, in doing so, I became very aware of the lack of writing on caesareans in general, and in particular, of the failure to address the psychological and emotional aspects of caesarean birth.[1] Consequently, our experiences as caesarean mothers remain unnamed and unspoken. One caesarean mother expressed this when she said:

We just don't have the words to say how we feel.

Another wrote:

I felt so . . . I don't even know how I felt. I have my wonderful beautiful baby, healthy, but. The 'but' is what I still don't quite understand.

I hope that in this book we will begin to find the words and to name our experience.

Much of what has been written about caesareans falls into one of two categories. There are those books that take a very gloomy outlook and assume that having a caesarean is always and inevitably a distressing and depressing experience. Then there are other books which assume that having a caesarean is always, or could always be, a highly satisfying and fulfilling alternative mode of childbirth. Neither approach fully reflects the reality of caesarean birth. Such approaches also fail to reflect the diversity of the caesarean experience. We all react to events in different ways and no two caesarean mothers will feel exactly the same about their birth experience. Even the same mother may feel very differently about a first and second caesarean birth.

Equally, the circumstances in which a caesarean birth takes place vary enormously. No two caesarean births are identical. A caesarean may be carried out for a number of different reasons. It may be planned months in advance or it may be carried out as an emergency procedure with only a few minutes warning. It may be carried out under general anaesthetic with the mother unconscious and the father pacing the corridor, or it may be performed with regional anaesthesia, like an epidural, with the mother awake and alert and her partner at her side. It may be a woman's first caesarean or it may be her fourth. It may be the culmination of a healthy, trouble-free pregnancy, or a pregnancy beset with problems. The caesarean may follow either a satisfying, or highly traumatic, vaginal birth. It may be a straightforward textbook caesarean. Alternatively, it may be accompanied by a number of debilitating complications. The mother may enter the operating theatre fully prepared and informed. Equally, she may know very little about caesarean birth and find the whole process bewildering.

We all hold different expectations about childbirth. Some women see it as an almost mystical experience whilst others expect it to be a terrible ordeal of relentless pain, and these perceptions will colour our experience of caesarean birth. Sometimes, the caesarean will be seen as a much needed life-saving operation, but in other situations caesareans are carried out for less clearcut reasons and a woman may be left questioning whether her caesarean was entirely necessary. Women and their partners may or may not feel involved and informed in the decision to carry out a caesarean and in the events that lead up to it. Women may receive ample care and support prior to, during and after a caesarean, or there may be a complete lack of such care and support. All of these things play a large part in determining the quality of our experience of caesarean birth and on the nature and extent of its emotional aftermath.

As well as being complex and varied, the caesarean experience also contains many contradictions. Childbirth has been described as a mixed blessing with the potential for enormously meaningful gain and tremendously disturbing loss.[2] Because of this, a caesarean birth may be remembered as both the best of times and the worst of times:

> I've tried to write about my experience a thousand times, but I just can't. So much happens and there's so much to it. It was heaven and it was hell all at once.

In writing this book I have tried to reflect the experiences of caesarean mothers (and fathers) in all their variety and complexity. It is clearly important to acknowledge the difficult feelings that a number of women feel after a caesarean and to document the negative side of caesarean birth. However, we also need to look at positive caesarean experiences, not only because many women do feel happy about having had a caesarean, but also because such experiences can tell us a lot about what we can do, as consumers of maternity care, and what health professionals involved in our care may do, to ensure that every woman's experience of caesarean childbirth is as positive as it may be.

Around 200 women took part in the research for this book by completing questionnaires and giving written accounts of their experiences and feelings. I contacted these women via requests in *Practical Parenting* magazine, in the newsletter of the Caesarean Support Network and in the National Childbirth Trust's journal, *New Generation*. The resulting questionnaires and accounts reflected a wide variety of experiences. The women ranged in age from 18 to 42; many had had two, three or even four caesareans; some wrote their accounts days or weeks after their caesareans, others wrote as much as ten years after the event; some summed up their feelings in a few lines, others wrote a dozen or more pages. All the women who took part had something important to say about their experience of caesarean childbirth.

Although this book is about the psychological experience of giving birth by caesarean, I have also included a substantial amount of medical information. There are two reasons why such information is of crucial importance, both to those facing a caesarean and to those who have had a caesarean. Firstly, all the evidence from health psychology suggests that clear and realistic information reduces fear before operations, enhances emotional well-being after surgery and may even promote faster physical recovery.[3] For those of you facing a caesarean, medical information can help to prepare you so that you will not be frightened or taken aback by the many medical procedures involved in caesarean birth. For those reading this book after having a caesarean, such information will help you to piece together all that has happened to you and why. Secondly, medical information is empowering. It enables us to take a more active role in childbearing decisions rather than being the passive recipients of medical opinion. This sense of empowerment can help us to sail through even the most difficult of birth experiences.

This book also contains some sociological perspectives on caesarean birth. We cannot divorce childbirth from its social context, for this social context is the backcloth to our experiences of caesarean birth. It will shape not only our expectations of caesarean birth, but also our response to it, the responses of those around us, the type and quality of care we receive, and even, in some instances, whether we have a caesarean delivery at all.

Finally, this book has a political purpose. As the users of the maternity services we have some power, both individually and collectively, to challenge current practices and to work towards a future in which all caesareans are necessary caesareans; in which each caesarean mother receives ample and appropriate care, support and information; and in which every woman who gives birth by caesarean feels emotionally strengthened rather than wounded, and emerges from the experience with her sense of self intact.

1   Why a Caesarean?

In Britain around 90,000 babies are born by caesarean every year, that is nearly 12 per cent of all births.[1] In America, a quarter of all babies enter the world this way. Caesarean birth rates in Canada and Australia are trailing just behind those of the USA; and throughout Europe increasing numbers of women are giving birth by caesarean.[2]

There are many different reasons for delivering a baby by caesarean. Sometimes the reasons are purely medical, but non-medical factors can also exert a strong influence on the decision to operate. Every caesarean mother needs to understand why her baby was born this way, if she is to assimilate and come to terms with the experience. As one caesarean mother wrote:

> Even now, two years on, I still have not had a real explanation as to why the caesarean was necessary. I think about it quite a lot.

To answer the question 'Why a caesarean?', I will begin by considering the medical reasons for caesarean birth. These are listed below with the most common reasons for performing a caesarean appearing near the top of the list. Some of the reasons are absolute indications for a caesarean, that is situations in which the only possible way of safely delivering the baby is by caesarean. Others are possible indications, where a caesarean is not always necessary and where medical professionals may disagree about whether this form of delivery is the best course of action.

DISPROPORTION

Disproportion, also referred to as fetopelvic or cephalopelvic disproportion or CPD, means that the baby is too large to fit through the mother's pelvis. This may be because the baby is large; because the mother's pelvis is smaller than average; or it may be due to a combination of these two reasons.

In most cases, the decision to carry out a caesarean for disproportion is undertaken after labour has begun. Signs that disproportion may be a factor include the baby's head remaining high and not descending into your pelvis, your cervix failing to dilate or dilating very slowly, or your baby becoming distressed during labour.

If your caesarean was carried out for suspected disproportion you may have an x-ray of your pelvis, known as x-ray pelvimetry, some time after the birth to help to confirm the diagnosis of disproportion. It is important to remember that if your first caesarean was carried out for disproportion, this does not necessarily mean that it will arise in any future pregnancies. The fit between a baby and a mother's pelvis depends not only on the size of the pelvis, but also on the size of the baby, his exact position and the extent to which the head moulds during labour. The size and shape of your pelvis can also alter during labour as the ligaments that join the pelvic bones stretch allowing the bones to move apart, and the position you adopt during this time can sometimes make all the difference since squatting can increase pelvic dimensions by up to 30 per cent.[3]

In some cases, disproportion is diagnosed during pregnancy. An internal examination during pregnancy is usually carried out to give a rough indication of the size of your pelvis. Your height and shoe size may also be noted; the shorter a woman is the more likely she is to have a small pelvis. This is not necessarily problematic since small women often have small babies, and 80 per cent of women under 5'3" (160 cm) tall go on to have vaginal deliveries.[4] It used to be thought that having small feet was a good means of determining a small pelvis, however recent evidence suggests that height is a better indication than shoe size.[5] Another sign that disproportion may be present is if your baby's head has not engaged — if it has not entered the pelvic cavity — in the last weeks of pregnancy. However, research suggests that the significance of non-engagement as a sign of disproportion has yet to be clearly established. [6]

If disproportion is a possibility you may be asked to have a pelvic x-ray towards the end of your pregnancy. Hospitals vary enormously in the extent to which pelvic x-rays are undertaken during pregnancy, and some have argued that there is no justification for antenatal x-ray pelvimetry, at least when the baby is lying in the usual head downwards position. [7] Although such x-rays can give some indication of how likely a vaginal delivery will be, they can rarely do so with sufficient accuracy to justify carrying out a caesarean just in case. For this reason, if it is your first pregnancy and disproportion is suspected, most obstetricians will advise you to have a trial of labour (where labour is allowed to progress naturally, but is carefully monitored and everything is ready should a caesarean become necessary) rather than an elective caesarean (one that is planned in advance).

FAILURE TO PROGRESS

Another common reason for a caesarean is failure to progress during labour, sometimes also referred to as prolonged labour or dystocia.

Sometimes labour fails to progress during the first stage, when the cervix does not dilate at the prescribed rate or within set time limits. There are many reasons for this. Firstly, it is important to realise that all biological processes vary among individuals and some of us will take longer to dilate than others without there being any underlying medical problem. It is also true that definitions of prolonged labour have altered over time so that an increasing number of women have labours that fall into this category. One particular event that imposes a time limit on labour is when the membranes have ruptured before labour has begun or early on in it. When membranes have been ruptured for over twenty-four hours there is a risk of infection that might affect the baby. Medical opinions differ about the most appropriate course of action if your membranes have been ruptured for this length of time: some will automatically carry out a caesarean, some will attempt to speed up labour using an oxytocin drip and others will watch carefully and only intervene when there are signs of infection, such as an increase in your temperature or changes in your heart rate or in your baby's heart rate.

One reason for failure to progress may be that your contractions are weak — this is more common in first labours, in women who have had four or more babies and in older first-time mothers. Another reason is disproportion. The baby's position can also affect the labour's progress. In addition, a number of non-medical factors can alter the length of labour: women who are left alone and unsupported during labour may have longer labours, and some studies have shown that providing continuous one-to-one support for labouring women has a significant effect in reducing the time it takes.[8] Similarly, both fear and changes in the environment have been shown to hold up labour.[9] It is not uncommon for a woman who is experiencing strong and regular contractions at home, to come into hospital and for her contractions to slow and become weak or even to stop altogether. There is also ample evidence to show that maternal position and mobility can affect length of labour. Being upright and walking around tend to shorten labour, whilst reclining in bed often prolongs it.[10]

If it is decided that labour is not progressing well, an intravenous drip containing oxytocin will usually be set up to accelerate the process. Often this will bring about progress to full dilation, but in some instances it does not achieve the desired result and a caesarean delivery becomes necessary. Other times, the use of oxytocin may lead to fetal distress, and a caesarean then becomes necessary.[11]

One particular reason for carrying out a caesarean is failed induction. Attempts to start off labour artificially are not always successful, particularly if your cervix has not yet softened in readiness for labour.[12] If induction fails, then your baby will need to be born by caesarean.

Sometimes failure to progress occurs during the second stage of labour, the pushing stage. This may be due to weak contractions; maternal exhaustion; disproportion; the presence of an anterior lip, that is where there is incomplete dilation and part of the cervix is holding back the baby's head; or malposition, where the baby is lying in an awkward position. Epidural anaesthesia is also known to prolong the length of the second stage.[13] When there is failure to progress during the second stage a forceps delivery will often be carried out. Or a ventouse vacuum extractor may be used as an alternative to forceps. When it is felt that an assisted vaginal delivery would be inadvisable, the baby will be born by caesarean. The decision about which course of action to take will depend upon a number of factors, including the suspected cause of the failure to progress, the exact position of the baby, how far the baby has descended, how experienced your doctor is in carrying out difficult forceps or ventouse deliveries and on his or her own beliefs about the relative safety of forceps and caesarean deliveries. Sometimes an attempt at a forceps or ventouse delivery fails and then a caesarean is the only alternative left.

FETAL DISTRESS

Fetal distress occurs when the baby is short of oxygen. Sometimes it is diagnosed before labour begins; more often, however, it occurs once labour is underway.

There are three main signs of fetal distress: changes in the baby's heart rate, meconium staining in the waters that surround the baby and changes in the pH balance of the baby's blood. During labour your baby's heart will be monitored, either intermittently by fetal stethoscope or hand-held ultrasound monitor (sonicaid), or continuously via monitors attached to a belt round your abdomen or via an electrode clipped onto your baby's scalp. A fetal heart rate that is consistently fast, for example over 160 beats per minute, or persistently slow, say less than 120 beats per minute, is thought to indicate that the baby may be lacking oxygen.[14] Babies heart rates tend to decrease in response to contractions then quickly return to normal. If your baby's heart rate takes a long time to recover after contractions then late decelerations are said to be occurring, which are also a sign of fetal distress. In some instances, changes in the baby's heart rate are severe and it is clear to all that an immediate caesarean is necessary to save the baby's life. Often, however, the heart rate changes are more ambiguous and false diagnoses of fetal distress can occur.

The second sign of fetal distress is the presence of meconium in the amniotic fluid that surrounds the baby. Meconium is the dark greeny-black substance that is the first contents of the baby's bowel. Meconium staining does not necessarily mean that your baby is in distress, but, particularly if the meconium is thick and profuse, it does indicate the condition of your baby needs to be very carefully monitored.

The most accurate way to determine the existence of fetal distress is fetal scalp blood sampling, where a small sample of blood is taken from your baby's head and its acidity and oxygen content is analysed. Some experts believe that the diagnosis of fetal distress should always be confirmed by taking a fetal blood sample in situations where a caesarean is proposed. However, this practice is not always carried out routinely when fetal distress is suspected because of the time-consuming nature of fetal blood sampling.

Women are often told that their caesarean was carried out because of fetal distress, yet they are left wondering what caused the baby to become distressed. The cause of fetal distress is often unknown, although sometimes the reason becomes apparent after the birth. It may be caused by the placenta not functioning well, the baby's umbilical cord being compressed or by disproportion. It may also occur because the cord is wrapped tightly around the baby's neck, particularly if the cord is unusually short or if it is wrapped round more than once. A sudden change in the force of the contractions can also precipitate fetal distress, such as when the membranes are ruptured[15] or when labour is accelerated with an oxytocin drip.[16] Lying on your back has also been shown to cause fetal distress in some cases, since in this position the weight of the uterus presses down on the large artery of the heart and reduces the blood flow to the uterus and placenta.[17] The lowering of maternal blood pressure that occurs when an epidural is set up has also been implicated in fetal distress in some instances.[18]

The action that is taken, should your baby become distressed, will depend on both the severity of the fetal distress and when it occurs. Fetal distress is sometimes mild, in which case labour may be allowed to proceed. Changes in your baby's heart rate may be transient and quickly return to normal. Fetal distress sometimes responds to simple measures such as a change in the mother's position. If your baby becomes distressed during the second stage of labour, a forceps or ventouse delivery or an episiotomy (a cut to enlarge the birth canal) may be performed to speed up the delivery. However, if fetal distress is persistent and moderate or severe, and vaginal delivery is not imminent, then your baby will need to be born by caesarean.

BREECH BABY

Around 3 per cent of babies are breech, that is they are lying in a bottom-down rather than a head-down position. A breech presentation is usually diagnosed during pregnancy. Before 32 weeks of pregnancy, around a quarter of all babies are breech, but the vast majority of these turn to the head down position of their own accord. Occasionally, a breech presentation is not diagnosed until labour is well underway.

Breech deliveries are seen as problematic because of the very small risk of the baby's head becoming trapped after the rest of the baby has been born. This is a possibility if the baby's bottom descends through a cervix that is not completely dilated, if there is some disproportion or if the baby's head is at an awkward angle or is unusually large. No one knows the exact extent of this risk and there has been much debate amongst obstetricians about the best way to manage breech deliveries. Consequently, the proportion of breech babies delivered by caesarean varies enormously from obstetrician to obstetrician, from hospital to hospital and from country to country.

Some obstetricians recommend that all breech babies be delivered by caesarean in first-time mothers. Some even go as far as to recommend universal caesarean delivery of breech babies. However, there is very little research evidence to support such policies.[19]

The more typical practice in Britain is to carry out a pelvic x-ray late in the pregnancy to determine the size of the mother's pelvis and a scan to indicate the size and position of the baby. If your pelvis is found to be average or above average in size, if the baby is predicted to be less than 8lbs (3.6 kg) in weight and if she is curled up in a ball with the neck flexed at the correct angle, you will be typically offered a trial of labour. If not, a caesarean will be recommended.

If you have a trial of labour you will be expected to make steady progress during labour. If your labour does not progress well you will be advised to have a caesarean.

When conditions for a trial of labour are favourable women are sometimes given the choice of whether to have a trial of labour or an elective caesarean. This is often a very difficult decision, especially given the way vaginal breech deliveries are typically managed. One woman said:

> Following x-rays I was told I had every chance of delivering 'normally'. 'Normally' meant on my back with my legs in stirrups, large episiotomy, forceps and preferably under epidural anaesthetic. I have always had two nightmares regarding childbirth and here I was being asked which of the two I wished to endure.

There are a few dissenting voices. Michel Odent, whose pioneering work at Pithiviers in France, has become internationally renowned, believes that so long as the first stage of labour progresses normally, then a natural vaginal delivery in the supported squatting position is the safest way to deliver all breech babies.[20]

There has also been a lot of debate about external version. This is when a doctor gently manipulates a woman's abdomen, during the last few weeks of pregnancy, in an attempt to turn a breech baby to a head-down position. This is not always successful — some babies refuse to be turned and others revert to breech after being turned. There are also some risks associated with external version: the placenta may become separated; in turning the baby the cord may become looped round the baby's neck; and, in some cases, it may cause premature labour. For these reasons external version is attempted less frequently nowadays than in the past, although it still has its advocates. The medical evidence appears to suggest that there are sound reasons for attempting to turn breech babies at term or during labour, when babies are more likely to remain head down once turned and when any complications that do arise can be remedied by carrying out an emergency caesarean.[21]

TRANSVERSE LIE

Transverse lie, also sometimes referred to as shoulder presentation, is when a baby is lying horizontally, neither head down nor bottom down. This position is quite unusual, occurring around ten times less frequently than breech presentations. Like breech babies, many babies lying in a transverse position will move into a head-down position of their own accord towards the end of pregnancy. There is no way that a baby in a transverse position can be born vaginally. In some cases, obstetricians will attempt to turn a transverse baby to a head down position. If this fails then your baby will need to be born by caesarean. In other cases, obstetricians may decide that an attempt at external version is unwarranted and an elective caesarean will be recommended.

MALPOSITION

When a baby is lying in a breech or transverse position, it is referred to as a malpresentation, since part of the baby other than the head is presenting. Malposition, however, occurs when a baby is lying in a head-down position, but its head is not in the ideal position. The three main types of malposition are occipito posterior, face and brow presentations. An elective caesarean is rarely carried out for malposition, since it often rights itself spontaneously during labour.

The most common type of malposition is the occipito posterior position, sometimes also referred to as face-to-pubis, when your baby is lying with her face pointing towards your abdomen and her spine against yours. Around 5 per cent of babies lie in this position at the onset of labour, and it is more common in first labours than in subsequent ones. If your baby is in a posterior position labour will tend to be longer and you may experience a lot of backache. Given enough time, the majority of posterior babies will spontaneously rotate to the more usual anterior position, with their back against the mother's abdominal wall, during labour. Occasionally, a posterior baby may remain posterior and be born vaginally, but this is unusual since a wider part of the baby's head must come though the mother's pelvis first. Sometimes a posterior baby can be turned using forceps. In some instances, however, posterior babies fail to descend sufficiently for a forceps delivery, or get stuck, and if this is the case, then your baby will need to be born by caesarean.

In around one in 300 labours it is the baby's face rather than the top of his head that is coming first, and this is known as a face presentation. If your baby is in this position a vaginal delivery is sometimes possible, but often a caesarean will be needed.

A brow presentation occurs when your baby's forehead rather than the top of her head is the part that is coming first. Brow presentations are rare, occurring in only around one in 1,000 deliveries. A baby cannot be born vaginally in this position, so, unless your baby takes up a more favourable position during labour, a caesarean delivery will be necessary.

Another situation that may necessitate a caesarean delivery is deep transverse arrest. This occurs when your baby's head descends in a sideways or lateral position and becomes stuck. It can sometimes be remedied with forceps or by hand, but if not your baby will have to be born by caesarean.

PREVIOUS CAESAREAN

A previous caesarean delivery is rarely, in itself, a sufficient reason for future births to be by caesarean. Whilst there is a very small risk of the old caesarean scar separating during labour, this separation is usually minor and of no consequence to mother or baby. In addition, the risks of scar separation are offset by the greater risks inherent in a caesarean delivery. Therefore, trial of labour is the logical choice unless there is a repeating or new indication for a caesarean delivery.[22] It is important to note however, that this may not apply to the minority of caesarean mothers who have classical (vertical) scars, since such scars are more prone to separate than the more common lower segment (bikini) variety. Also, if separation does occur in a classical scar this is usually more serious and dangerous than if it happens with a lower segment scar. Consequently, although it is not unheard of for women with classical scars to go on to have vaginal deliveries, most obstetricians will recommend an elective caesarean in this situation.

Despite the fact that all the medical evidence points to the relative safety of trials of labour for the majority of caesarean mothers, and despite the fact that in Europe, unlike in the USA, there has never been strict adherence to the outdated dictum 'once a caesarean, always a caesarean', around half of all caesarean mothers in Britain will go on to have future deliveries by caesarean. Clearly, this cannot be due to repeating or new reasons for caesarean delivery arising in every case. There are a number of other reasons why caesarean mothers are more likely to have subsequent deliveries by caesarean.

Firstly, when a woman has had one caesarean the threshold for carrying out a caesarean in future pregnancies tends to alter. So, for example, if situations arise which are not, in themselves, indications for a caesarean, such as slightly raised blood pressure, the baby not being in the ideal position or being a few days overdue, a caesarean may be recommended if a woman has already had one, when it would not be in other cases. In addition, if you have had one caesarean and there are no new or repeating indications for a caesarean delivery, you may well be given the choice of whether to have an elective caesarean or a trial of labour. Then you will have to make the sometimes difficult decision of whether to go for a trial of labour which may result in a vaginal birth, but which may also result in an emergency caesarean, which may need to be under general anaesthetic, or whether to go for an elective caesarean, where at least you know what will happen and where you will have the option of being awake for the birth. In weighing up the relative merits of each course of action, many women decide on an elective caesarean. If you have had two or more caesareans, most obstetricians would strongly advise you to have future births by caesarean for this reason alone. However, there have been a number of recent research papers supporting the relative safety of trials of labour after two or more caesareans.[23] So there would appear to be some grounds for challenging the common practice of scheduling repeat caesareans after two previous caesareans.

Finally, the way in which trials of labour after a previous caesarean are typically conducted — with short time limits and quite high levels of medical intervention — may mean that women who might otherwise have gone on to give birth vaginally end up having a caesarean. All these issues are discussed in greater detail in Chapter 9.

PLACENTA PRAEVIA

In placenta praevia the placenta (afterbirth) is lying low down so that it is covering or partially covering the lower part of the uterus. This occurs in around one in 200 pregnancies. A vaginal delivery is not possible in most cases of placenta praevia because the baby's exit is blocked or partially blocked, and even if the baby could make her way out there would inevitably be bleeding from the placental site which is dangerous to both mother and baby. There are, however, different degrees of placenta praevia and very occasionally where the placenta praevia is very marginal, a vaginal delivery may be possible.

The main signs of placenta praevia are bright red, painless bleeding, usually late in pregnancy or more rarely during labour, and malpresentation, such as breech or transverse lie. Since women now typically have a routine ultrasound scan during pregnancy, most cases of placenta praevia are detected at this earlier stage and an elective caesarean is planned. It is important to realise, nevertheless, that if a scan in early or mid-pregnancy reveals a low-lying placenta, which around 5 per cent of scans at this stage do, this does not necessarily mean that you have placenta praevia and will need a caesarean. In the vast majority of cases, the placenta will move upwards to a more normal position during the course of pregnancy. If a low-lying placenta is detected, you will be re-scanned towards the end of pregnancy to see if this is so or if you have placenta praevia.

ANTEPARTUM HAEMORRHAGE

In around 6 per cent of pregnancies women experience some

bleeding in the last twelve weeks of pregnancy. This is known as an antepartum haemorrhage. The bleeding may be slight and last only a short while before stopping of its own accord or it may be severe and persistent. In around half of all cases of antepartum haemorrhage the cause of the bleeding is not known and is classified as bleeding of uncertain origin. Most of the remaining cases are due to either placenta praevia or placental abruption.

Placental abruption is when the placenta begins to come away from the wall of the uterus. It is sometimes, but not always, accompanied by bleeding and abdominal pain. It is often not known why placental abruption occurs, but it is more common in women who have had four or more children and may occur after some sort of trauma, such as a blow to the abdomen.

In mild cases of antepartum haemorrhage, which are of uncertain origin or due to mild placental abruption, your condition and that of your baby will be watched carefully and, if all is well, pregnancy and delivery can proceed as usual. If, however, the haemorrhage is moderate or severe, your baby will need to be born quickly, and in most cases this will mean a caesarean birth.

PROLAPSED CORD

In around one in 300 of all deliveries the baby's umbilical cord slips past the baby down into the vagina when the waters break. This can happen when there is not a close fit between the part of the baby that is coming first and the cervix. Therefore prolapsed cord is more likely to occur with very small or premature babies, or when there is a malpresentation, such as breech or transverse lie, or a malposition, such as an occipito posterior position. A prolapsed cord is a dire emergency because the cord is likely to become compressed between the baby and the mother's bony pelvis, precipitating severe fetal distress. In addition, the cord is very sensitive and merely being touched or becoming cold could make its arteries go into spasm, cutting off the baby's supply of oxygen. If the cord prolapses and your cervix is dilated or nearly dilated, an immediate forceps or ventouse delivery may be possible, otherwise an emergency caesarean will be carried out. You will be placed on a trolley with your head lower than your pelvis and a midwife or doctor may attempt to hold the baby off the cord as you are rushed to the operating theatre.

VULNERABLE BABIES

Sometimes a caesarean will be carried out because the baby is in a vulnerable state and it is felt that he would not stand up well to a vaginal delivery.

If it appears that your baby is not growing very well, which may be referred to as interuterine growth retardation, or being small-for-dates, it may be decided that she would be better out than in. If this is so she might be induced. However, some obstetricians believe that such babies, whose health may already be compromised, are likely to be more safely delivered by caesarean.

Another category of vulnerable babies are those that are born prematurely. There has been much debate surrounding the issue of whether premature babies should be delivered vaginally or by caesarean. Before the advent of sophisticated neonatal care facilities, the chances of a very premature baby surviving were so low that performing a caesarean was rarely justifiable. Nowadays, the likelihood that a premature baby will survive is much greater and caesarean delivery is much more likely to be considered as an option. Some studies have shown that premature babies fare better when delivered by caesarean, and this is particularly so for very low birth-weight babies and for breech babies.[24] However, such studies have been criticised for not comparing like with like, and some experts have argued that considering the lack of reliable evidence about the benefits of caesarean delivery to the premature baby, and with its known risks to the mother, caesarean delivery for premature babies should be the exception rather than the rule.[25] In the absence of randomised controlled trials we simply do not know which is the safest type of delivery for premature babies.

Twins are often classified as vulnerable babies since there is a tendency for them to be small and to have a premature delivery.

Although a twin pregnancy is certainly not an absolute indication for a caesarean birth, twins are more commonly delivered by caesarean than single babies for reasons of size and prematurity, and because there are sometimes difficulties in delivering the second twin. It is also true that in around half of twin pregnancies at least one baby will be breech, and, as discussed above, this may be an indication for a caesarean delivery. It is currently common practice for triplets to be routinely delivered by caesarean, but in at least one study this policy has been questioned and vaginal delivery for some sets of triplets is recommended. [26]

Finally, a caesarean delivery is sometimes recommended for so-called special babies, that is babies who are the result of years of treatment for infertility, or babies conceived after a previous stillbirth.

PROBLEMS IN THE MOTHER

There are a number of problems affecting the pregnant woman's health that may indicate that a caesarean birth is the best course of action. One of the most common problems is pre-eclampsia. The main symptoms of pre-eclampsia include high blood pressure, protein in your urine and water retention. It is a serious condition which, if untreated, can result in fits that are dangerous to both mother and baby. The usual treatment is bed rest and sometimes drugs to lower blood pressure, but if these measures fail to resolve the problem it will be necessary for your baby to be born without much delay. Sometimes it will be possible to induce the baby, but in other cases, particularly if the pre-eclampsia is severe, he will need to be born by caesarean.

Diabetes is another condition that has traditionally been associated with caesarean birth. Diabetic women tend to have large babies, and because of this, disproportion, and hence caesarean delivery is more likely. However, in recent years, there have been enormous advances in the treatment of diabetes in pregnancy, and where diabetes is well controlled, caesarean delivery can often be avoided.

If you suffer from genital herpes, the herpes virus could be transferred to your baby during a vaginal delivery and this can be very dangerous to a newborn baby. This can only happen, however, if the herpes is active at the time of delivery. Therefore, you will be tested towards the end of your pregnancy and if the virus is active an elective caesarean will be necessary, if it is not a vaginal delivery may be possible.

If you have had previous surgery on your uterus, such as an operation to remove fibroids, you may be advised to have an elective caesarean because of the small risk of the old scar separating. Whether a caesarean is recommended or whether a vaginal delivery may be possible will depend on the extent of the surgery, the position of the scar and whether the uterine cavity was entered during the operation. If you have had previous surgery to your vagina, such as an operation to repair a vaginal prolapse, then you will invariably be advised to have an elective caesarean to prevent damage to the repair. Similarly, if you suffered a particularly bad tear or episiotomy in a previous delivery, especially one that required resuturing, you may be offered the option of a caesarean in future deliveries.

Other health problems that may necessitate a caesarean delivery include low-lying fibroids or cysts that would get in the way of a vaginal delivery. Women suffering from heart disease may also be advised to have a caesarean. However, with the use of an epidural and forceps it is often possible for women with heart disease to give birth vaginally without undue stress on the heart.

Women who have their first baby in their late thirties or early forties have a slightly increased risk of needing a caesarean delivery. Whilst maternal age alone is never a sufficient reason for carrying out a caesarean, occasionally, when combined with other factors, being an older first-time mother may tip the balance in favour of a caesarean birth.

THE RISING CAESAREAN BIRTH RATE

It would be nice to think that medical necessity was the sole determining criteria for carrying out a caesarean. But the enormous variation in the numbers of caesarean births that take place in different countries suggests that this cannot be the case. In the USA there is what can only be described as an epidemic of caesareans. One in 4 American babies are born by caesarean, and caesarean section is now the most commonly performed operation in America.[27] In some hospitals in Brazil as many as 75 per cent of babies enter the world this way.[28] Other countries such as Canada, Australia and Singapore, have caesarean rates that are approaching those of the USA.[29] In Europe rates vary between 4 and 12 per cent.[30] Some of the lowest rates are found in the Netherlands, Czechoslovakia and the Republic of Ireland where the percentage of babies born by caesarean remains well within single figures.

In Britain, nearly 12 per cent of all babies are born by caesarean. Yet this figure masks considerable variations between regions and hospitals. At least one National Health Service hospital has reported a caesarean section rate of 25 per cent,[31] and some private hospitals are reputed to have rates of around 40 per cent.[32] As in the rest of the world, there has been a substantial rise in the proportion of babies delivered by caesarean. In 1960 around 3 per cent of babies were born in this way; by 1970 this figure had risen to around 5 per cent. A steep rise during the 1970s meant that by 1980 the caesarean birth rate reached nearly 10 per cent. Rates have continued to rise, albeit at a slower rate, to stand at over 11 per cent in England and Wales, and nearly 14 per cent in Scotland, in 1985 and 1988 respectively, the most recent years for which figures are available.

Some of this rise is justifiable on medical grounds. It is certainly true that caesarean birth has become safer in recent years, with improvements in antibiotics, in anaesthesia and in surgical techniques. This means that the risks of not performing a caesarean will outweigh the risks of performing one in a growing number of cases. Many would claim that the greater numbers of breech and premature babies being delivered by caesarean, and the greater tendency to resort to caesarean rather than difficult forceps delivery, are the major factors behind the rise in caesareans. It has also been suggested that the increased tendency for women to delay childbearing until a later age is partly responsible for the rising numbers of caesarean births. Furthermore, it should be noted that a rise in the caesarean rate tends to have a knock-on effect and to fuel further rises, because a woman who has one baby by caesarean is more likely to have caesareans in future deliveries than if she had had a vaginal birth in the first instance. These growing numbers are also self-perpetuating because of the resultant loss of clinical skills: as the caesarean rate rises, skills such as vaginal breech delivery, external version and difficult forceps delivery, are lost or fail to be acquired.

It is often claimed that the rise in caesarean rates is mainly due to modern obstetrics saving the lives of large numbers of babies who would have otherwise died. Whilst it is true that a caesarean is often a life-saving operation, to attribute decreases in perinatal mortality, that is in babies dying at or around birth, to the increased use of caesarean delivery is misleading. The exact relationship between caesarean section rates and perinatal mortality is unclear. For example, in Ireland during the period from 1965 to 1980, the caesarean rate remained virtually unchanged at less than 5 per cent, but perinatal mortality fell by more than half.[33] Similarly, the USA, which has one of the highest caesarean rates in the world, has poor perinatal mortality statistics compared with Europe where fewer caesareans are carried out.[34]

There has been much debate about what the ideal rate for caesarean births is. Obstetrician Peter Hungtingford believes there is cause for concern if the caesarean rate rises above 6 per cent.[35] Similarly, Wendy Savage believes that there is no justification for a national caesarean rate of more than 6 to 8 per cent.[36] Likewise, other researchers have concluded that there is little improvement in the health of newborns or mothers when caesarean rates rise above 7 per cent.[37]

It is apparent, then, that current rates are being driven upwards by something other than clearly defined medical need. Indeed, epidemiologist Jonathan Lomas and Professor of Obstetrics Murray Enkin state that, 'The extent to which . . . non-medical determinants influence the observed operative delivery rates cannot be exactly calculated, but it is likely to be as great or greater than the influence of medical indications'.[38] Perhaps we should not be surprised that the way we give birth is influenced by non-medical considerations, for as researcher Colin Francome has pointed out, 'No human activity, including medical practice, is likely to be determined entirely on rational grounds.'[39]

Nevertheless, the realisation that in Britain every year there may be as many as 35,000 unnecessary or avoidable caesareans is both shocking and intolerable.[40]

NON-MEDICAL FACTORS

Defensive medicine is one of the main non-medical factors implicated in the rise in caesarean births. Defensive medicine is the practice of carrying out medical procedures not on medical grounds but rather on the grounds that in doing so doctors may avoid the risk of being sued for negligence. Although defensive medicine is probably less common in Britain than it is in the USA, over 80 per cent of British medical practitioners admit that they sometimes adopt practices simply to avoid negligence claims.[41] Defensive medicine is thought to arise in all areas of medicine, but it is said to be particularly rife in the field of obstetrics. In one study defensive medicine was the second most common reason given by obstetricians for the rise in caesarean births.[42] As one obstetrician wrote, 'The reason that the caesarean section rate is going up is that we're all scared stiff of litigation.'[43]

One case which many feel has had a significant influence on the practice of defensive obstetrics is the case of baby Whitehouse versus Jo Jordan. Baby Whitehouse suffered brain damage after an unsuccessful attempt at a forceps delivery by obstetrician Jo Jordan. The baby was awarded £100,000 in damages. However, Mr Jordan successfully appealed against the judgement, the award was set aside after two more judicial hearings and Jordan's decision to attempt a forceps delivery was vindicated. In the wake of this case, however, many obstetricians have become reluctant to attempt difficult forceps deliveries and tend to deliver by caesarean in such situations.

The use of continuous electronic monitoring with its permanent trace has also been implicated in defensive obstetrics and the rise in caesareans. It is suggested that some obstetricians believe they must deliver by caesarean whenever the baby's heart trace shows evidence of fetal distress, for fear that this trace will be used as evidence against them should the baby later prove to be mentally handicapped and despite their knowledge that only a few babies born by caesarean for fetal distress are actually in trouble. [44]

It has also been suggested that some caesareans are carried out for the convenience of the obstetrician. This is felt to be particularly true with regard to repeat caesareans. [45] One obstetrician has put forward the view that the reason for the rise in the caesarean rate is 'patience, rather than patients'. [46] He related how he had recently carried out a vaginal delivery at 5.30 a.m. after a long labour and speculated that many would have done a caesarean section at 11.30 p.m. for 'failure to progress'.

Staff shortages may also play a role. A number of obstetricians have commented that their heavy workload leaves them with little time on the labour ward to supervise difficult cases, and suggested that the junior staff were opting for caesarean deliveries where the presence of a more experienced consultant might have resulted in a vaginal birth. [47] Indeed, studies have shown that the decision to perform a caesarean is usually undertaken by junior medical staff and that in a third of cases consultants reviewing case notes at a later date stated that their decisions would have differed from those made by the junior staff. [48] Shortages of nursing staff may also contribute to the increase in the number of caesareans being performed. At least one obstetrician reported sometimes having to resort to caesarean delivery sooner rather than later because the shortage of qualified nursing staff meant that if he adopted a wait-and-see policy there might be no one available to assist at the operation should a caesarean later prove necessary. [49]

Another important factor is the type of stance taken in medicine. Is medicine practised in an aggressive, interventionist way, or is a more conservative, wait-and-see approach the norm? In the USA, the epidemic of caesareans may well be a reflection of the aggressive nature of American medicine in general, where rates of all types of surgery are more than twice those in Britain. [50] In obstetrics, it has been suggested that one of the major factors underlying the variations in caesarean rates, both internationally and within one country, is the dichotomy between interventionist practitioners, who like to manage and control every aspect of a woman's labour and to intervene routinely just in case something goes wrong, and conservative practitioners, who watch carefully and wait, only intervening when the need arises. [51] Some obstetricians claim that the highly interventionist approach, known as the active management of labour, is associated with low caesarean rates. The active management of labour (not to be confused with active birth) involves artificially rupturing the membranes once a woman is diagnosed as being in labour, and then using oxytocin to speed up labour if the cervix dilates at a rate of less than 1 cm per hour. However, this is a controversial issue. The limited medical evidence available to date suggests that active management does not lower caesarean rates, and its liberal use cannot be justified.[52] To intervene in a normal labour is not a benign action, since labour is a finely tuned physiological process and attempts to alter it may have deleterious effects on both mother and baby. Indeed, midwife-researcher Mary Renfew has described routine intervention in normal labour as being like using a sledgehammer to open the most delicate of containers.[53]

Routine forms of intervention include the withholding of food from labouring women, the artificial rupture of membranes, the expectation that women should adopt a semi-reclining position during labour, the use of continuous electronic monitoring, the use of oxytocin to accelerate normal labours that are progressing at a slower than average rate and induction solely on the grounds that a woman is a set number of days past her due date. All these practices may have a deleterious effect on labour, thereby necessitating further intervention and possibly a caesarean delivery — a process known as the 'cascade of intervention'.[54]

Continuous electronic monitoring is one form of intervention that has been specifically implicated in the rise in the number of caesareans being carried out. There are two main problems with routine continuous electronic monitoring. Firstly, in some cases, it may actually produce the fetal distress that it is designed to detect. This is because it tends to immobilise women and to restrict the positions they may adopt, which may precipitate fetal distress, and also make labour last longer. Where monitoring is internal, artificial rupture of membranes is necessary, and this procedure is also thought to increase the likelihood of fetal distress. The second problem is that heart rate tracings are notoriously difficult to interpret. They may be interpreted differently, not only by different obstetricians, but also by the same obstetrician at a later time.[55] Worryingly, the routine use of continuous monitoring has consistently been shown to double the caesarean rate.[56] This might well be acceptable if this type of monitoring helped to save babies' lives, but this does not appear to be the case. In all the randomised controlled trials that have been carried out to compare continuous and intermittent monitoring, intermittent monitoring was found to be as effective in preventing neonatal death, problems at birth and long-term impairment as continuous electronic monitoring.[57]

Another interesting perspective comes from obstetrician Wendy Savage, who believes that one important reason for the rise in the caesarean rate is that labour is being pushed on too fast.[58] She cites evidence that, in women having their first babies, twelve to twenty-four hours is the optimal length of labour, whereas many obstetricians like to see labour completed in less than twelve hours. If the labour cannot be speeded up to meet this time limit, some will resort to a caesarean delivery. Similarly, it is common practice for labour to be defined as abnormal if the rate of cervical dilation is less than 1 cm per hour once labour has become established, whereas the medical evidence suggests that a rate of 0.5 cm per hour may be a more appropriate lower limit.[59]

Taking a broader perspective, some have argued that the rise in caesareans represents the culmination of the historical trend of men taking over the process of birth from women. In caesarean childbirth, the male obstetrician, in one sense, acquires the female power of giving birth, and retains control of a process in which he cannot otherwise participate.[60] Labour is a process with its own powerful momentum and each labour is unique. It has been suggested that male obstetricians sometimes feel very uneasy dealing with events over which they have no control, and that they subsequently resort to interventions — including the ultimate intervention, caesarean birth — to quell this feeling of powerlessness and to retain some sense of control.[61]

It can also be argued that some male obstetricians find the powerful emotions of labour and childbirth very difficult to handle. This is evident in the comments of obstetrician Alan Smith, who, in attempting to defend high caesarean section rates, wrote, 'No woman these days has a labour of over fifteen hours without her or her consort becoming agitated, let alone the midwife and junior medical staff.'[62] He seems to be implying that the entry of a new baby into the world should be marked with as little emotion as a trip to the hairdressers. But these obstetricians, who would carry out caesareans to rescue us from the powerful emotions that long or difficult labour can bring, do not see the more profound and longer-lasting distress that may follow a caesarean birth that is perceived to be unnecessary.

Some people have argued that discussion of these broader, non-medical reasons for carrying out a caesarean has no place in a book aimed at caesarean mothers.[63] I believe, on the contrary, that it is essential for every woman whose baby is born by caesarean, to come to an understanding of why this was so. For many of us, the medical reasons discussed in the first half of this chapter are all that we will need to come to such an understanding. In other cases, however, we need to consider some of the wider issues that lie behind the statistics in order to find our own answers to the question 'Why a caesarean?'

2 The Easy Way to Have a Baby?

The way we experience caesarean birth is coloured, to a greater or lesser extent, by society's ideas about childbirth in general, and about caesarean birth in particular. These ideas influence both our own expectations of caesarean birth, and the responses of those around us — partners, friends, relations and medical professionals. Few of these beliefs are based on medical facts about caesareans and some of them are contradictory. Often there is a mismatch between our own experiences and society's ideas about caesarean birth. It is important to look at these ideas and beliefs in order to come to a full understanding of the caesarean experience.

One of the most widely held views about caesarean birth is that it is the easy way to have a baby. These caesarean mothers commented:

> The hardest part I have found is trying to explain my feelings to non-caesarean mothers who seem to see no problem — its easier and less painful in their eyes, so why worry.

> Hurtful comments such as 'A caesarean — that's the easy way to have a baby' didn't make me feel any better. Even my own GP said this to me.

The belief that a caesarean delivery is childbirth the easy way does not appear to come from facts about caesarean birth itself, but rather from deeply rooted fears about vaginal childbirth. Many people have been brought up with the ingrained biblical belief that women are cursed to bring forth children in sorrow and pain. Furthermore, when childbirth is portrayed on television and in films it is typically depicted as an agonising ordeal — images that we absorb from childhood onwards. Even educational films can portray vaginal birth in a very negative way.

One of the films most frequently used in schools is described as follows: 'The camera moved from the woman's agonized face to show the head of the baby forcing its way out of her vagina. There was blood as her perineum tore, and a passing shot of scissors.'[1] After watching this film several girls asked why all babies could not be delivered by caesarean.[2] Perhaps most of us grow up with a fear of the pain of labour and a dread of episiotomies or tears to the vagina. When vaginal birth is perceived in this way, caesarean birth may well appear as the easy option, since, in elective caesareans at least, labour pain and episiotomies or tears are avoided.

A PAIN-FREE DELIVERY?

Caesarean birth is often assumed to be pain-free, but this is rarely true. In the majority of cases, the decision to carry out a caesarean is made after labour has begun, sometimes after a long and painful labour. On top of this, caesarean mothers invariably have to cope with some degree of post-operative pain. Although the amount of pain experienced varies enormously from woman to woman, for the majority of us recovering from a caesarean is certainly not pain-free.

The view that caesarean birth is relatively painless is reinforced by magazine articles that sometimes fail to mention post-operative pain at all,[3] by books that speak of being 'uncomfortable for a few days'[4] and by doctors who tell us that we will feel 'a bit sore afterwards'. Such approaches may reassure us during pregnancy but ultimately they do us a disservice and leave us unprepared and taken aback by the mismatch between our expectations and our experience:

> I was aware of the most awful pain in my stomach, and couldn't understand why. I wondered if something had gone terribly wrong. I honestly hadn't realised I would be in pain!

GREAT EXPECTATIONS

The belief that vaginal birth is a dreadful ordeal and that caesarean birth is the easy option is certainly widespread, but resting somewhat awkwardly alongside this is the growing and opposing viewpoint which one caesarean mother refers to as the 'glorification of natural childbirth'. From this standpoint, vaginal birth which is free of all forms of medical intervention is revered and is seen as the only type of happy and fulfilling birth experience. Caesarean birth is perceived as the ultimate catastrophe. Yet few of us, however difficult our caesarean experiences, appreciate having the birth of our children likened to some kind of disaster:

> I feel that too little is written about caesareans, but we are overwhelmed with information about how to achieve natural birth without even a painkiller, never mind an operation! It's almost as if to have a caesarean is to be a failure, a secondrate birth and one to be swept under the carpet.

Ideas about vaginal birth — whether it is seen as an agonizing trial or the ultimate female experience — will not only shape the responses of those around us but will also colour our own expectations. Often it is those who had the greatest expectations of vaginal birth who are hit the hardest when the birth turns out to be a caesarean:

> Whilst pregnant I very much favoured natural childbirth. I wanted to give birth without pain relief and take an active role in the birth of my baby. I had read with great emotion the wonderful feelings of elation and achievement mothers felt after their baby's births. After the caesarean I felt devastated; I felt cheated of the birth. I also felt that I was a failure, not a proper mum, that all the months of expectation and preparation had led to the most awful experience of my life.

However, there is no reason to believe, as many do, that the main cause of unhappiness following a caesarean is that women expect too much of childbirth nowadays. From the many accounts of caesarean experiences I have received, it is apparent that what often upsets women most is not the fact that their babies were born by caesarean, but the way they were treated — the lack of care during labour or birth, being given no explanations or information, interventions being carried out without warning and without consent, unfeeling comments and not receiving adequate help and support during the hospital stay. Whilst it is important that every pregnant woman realises that in all births there is a chance that medical intervention will be necessary, no woman should expect to be treated in this way. The appropriate response to such treatment is anger, which we can use productively to fight for the sort of care birthing women deserve, not reproach for our high expectations of childbirth.

A HEALTHY MOTHER AND BABY ARE ALL THAT MATTERS?

Another common belief about caesarean birth, and one with which most caesarean mothers will be familiar, is that so long as mother and baby emerge from the experience alive and well this is all that matters. These women wrote:

> All too often any ill-feeling is brushed aside with 'as long as mother and baby are both safe, that's the main thing'.

> I suffered depression and a terrible guilt feeling of failure for a long time. When you explain to people this feeling you always get 'Well, it's worth it to see your son fit and healthy.' I'm not ungrateful for that but it wears a bit thin after a while. What about how I feel?

Of course it is of paramount importance to any expectant mother that her child is delivered alive and healthy. We are all grateful for our healthy babies. However, it is important to stress that, although this is the thing that matters most, it is not the only thing that matters. If a woman's experience of childbirth is such that it leaves her feeling violated and deeply depressed, this may well have a negative effect on her baby's well-being and development. But women's emotional pain is also important in its own right. The idea that a healthy mother and baby are all that matters may leave us believing that we are not entitled to feel any distress or sense of loss, that such feelings are selfish and self-indulgent. Yet acknowledging and accepting our feelings is a crucial step in the process of coming to terms with a difficult caesarean birth.

IT'S ALL IN THE HANDS OF THE DOCTORS?

Another common misconception about caesarean birth is that it is primarily a medical procedure and is therefore largely the concern of doctors rather than women themselves. The main way in which this belief manifests itself is in the lack of antenatal preparation for caesarean birth. Some books on pregnancy and childbirth make no mention of caesarean birth whatsoever,[5] others relegate it to a separate appendix at the back of the book[6] and the remainder tend to devote barely a page to the topic. Consequently, few of us feel adequately prepared or informed when we give birth by caesarean.

Not only do pregnancy books fail to discuss caesarean birth at any length, they also seldom depict it. Unlike the numerous, detailed, colour photographs of women giving birth vaginally that are found in most books on childbirth, images of caesarean birth are few and far between. If caesareans are depicted at all, the photographs are usually in black and white and rarely show the birth itself. When I came across the only close-up colour photograph I have seen of a baby being born by caesarean I was completely struck by this image and remained transfixed by it for a long time. It was an image with which I was totally unfamiliar, and yet this was the way my baby entered the world.

Caesarean birth also tends not to be covered in antenatal classes or it is mentioned only briefly before passing on to some other topic. Sometimes this unwillingness to discuss caesareans stems from concern about worrying those who go on to have vaginal births:

> When I asked the midwife who was taking the classes she said, 'We don't like to talk about it, you'll frighten the others.' I was really annoyed. I was frightened too!

It may also stem from the mistaken belief that in discussing caesarean birth an antenatal teacher may damage pregnant women's belief in their body's natural ability to give birth. Obviously there is a delicate line to tread between presenting childbirth as a normal healthy process and preparing those women whose births do not turn out to be straightforward, but I believe it is possible and certainly desirable to achieve this balance.

Doctors and midwives also appear to be reluctant to talk about caesarean birth when it is not an absolute certainty that one will be necessary:

> I asked quite a few times during my pregnancy about the possibility of having a caesarean, but the midwife seemed to ignore my question as if to say 'We will see what happens'.

> My baby was breech and I was scheduled for a trial of labour. I said that I would like to discuss what would be involved in a caesarean delivery in case this should prove necessary, but was told to 'go home and try not to think about it'.

When information is forthcoming we do not always take in what is offered. We do not imagine, or do not want to imagine, that a caesarean is something that might happen to us, so we skip over the relevant pages in pregnancy books and mentally switch off when it is mentioned in antenatal classes:

> I'd been to all the classes, and to be quite honest, I simply switched off when the thought of a caesar was mentioned, I think we all did. I just thought I wouldn't need one.

As a result of this lack of information and our own reluctance to face the possibility that a caesarean delivery may be necessary, most of us enter the operating theatre ill-prepared for what is to follow.

YOU'LL FEEL LIKE ANY OTHER MOTHER?

Despite the fact that it is perceived in largely medical terms, caesarean birth is not generally seen as the major operation that it is. We are told, 'Apart from the discomfort of the incision, a mother who has had a caesarean section can expect to recover from the birth of her baby in the same way as a mother who has had a vaginal delivery.'[7] Yet a caesarean section is major abdominal surgery, and after all such operations a period of convalescence is necessary. In addition, most patients who have undergone surgery have ample time to rest and recuperate, unlike caesarean mothers who have a new baby to care for. It is not therefore surprising that, in reality, many of us do take longer to recover from the birth than those who have given birth vaginally. Before we experience caesarean childbirth ourselves, we too may perceive caesareans in this way, and may be taken aback when it becomes apparent that caesarean birth is indeed a major operation. This caesarean mother said:

> I'd had no idea I would be checked throughout the night for blood pressure and temperature, etc. I was so green, despite reading countless pregnancy books and attending two sets of antenatal classes. All the caesarean mums were put in priority beds right beside the nurses, and treated extremely carefully. We were given stools to climb in and out of bed, and given the best chairs for breastfeeding, and loads of painkillers. It was quite incredible — I hadn't expected any of it. I suppose I thought I'd just jump up from the operating table with my baby and waltz off down the corridor with a few stitches!

The people around us often forget that we have had a major operation, and tend to assume that we are recovered as soon as the stitches have been removed. From then on, we are typically expected to cope as well as non-caesarean mothers:

> There were some totally insensitive friends who didn't understand why I wasn't leaping around the house and baking cakes.

A RISK-FREE DELIVERY?

The final common belief about caesarean birth is that it is the risk-free way to have a baby. This misconception appears to be held not only by the general public, but also by many in the medical profession.[8] Some obstetricians are even willing to carry out caesareans when there is no medical reason for doing so, simply because the mother requests a caesarean.[9] In doing so they are putting the health of both mother and baby at risk.

Whilst it is extremely rare nowadays for a woman to die as a result of caesarean childbirth, the risk is still considerably higher — sometimes as much as ten times higher — than that associated with vaginal birth.[10] Whilst some deaths are caused by the condition that necessitated the caesarean, at least half are thought to be caused by the operation itself.[11] This risk stems largely, but not solely, from complications with anaesthesia. Although elective caesareans are safer than emergency ones, maternal mortality is still between two and four times greater with an elective caesarean delivery than with a vaginal delivery.[12] Caesarean mothers also suffer more maternal morbidity, that is complications such as infection and haemorrhage, than vaginally delivered mothers. Around one in 5 women will suffer from a high temperature or fever following a caesarean delivery, usually caused by infection.[13] Infection can occur in the caesarean wound itself, in the chest, in the urinary tract and in the lining of the uterus. In one study almost half of all caesarean mothers suffered some form of complication.[14] Once a woman has given birth by caesarean, there is a greater chance that future deliveries will be by caesarean, and the small risk of scar separation. In addition to this, some research suggests that a woman's chances of becoming pregnant are somewhat lower after a caesarean than after a vaginal delivery.[15]

Few people are aware that caesarean delivery also presents risks to the baby. There is a tendency to assume that labour and vaginal birth put a baby under terrible stress. Indeed the 'hazards of the birth canal' are thought to be deeply embedded in obstetrical belief.[16] Whilst it is true that a small number of babies do not stand up to labour well and benefit greatly from caesarean delivery, this is not the case for the majority of babies. Babies are designed to be born vaginally. Contractions and the passage through the birth canal are said to benefit babies by squeezing out excess fluid from their lungs and by massaging the baby which helps to stimulate his or her breathing after birth.[17] Consequently babies born by caesarean are more likely to suffer from respiratory distress, that is difficulty in breathing, at birth.[18] In elective caesareans, there is also the risk that a baby will inadvertently be delivered prematurely, since methods for determining gestational age are not infallible.

There is no such thing as a risk-free delivery. It is a question of the balance of risks. Where there are definite medical reasons for carrying out a caesarean, the balance of risks strongly favours caesarean delivery. In the absence of such reasons, to carry out a caesarean delivery is to incur unnecessary risk. Some have argued that women have the right to decide to take this risk, and this may indeed be true. But it is essential that such decisions are made with full knowledge of the known risks, and not on the basis of the common misconception that a caesarean delivery is risk-free (nor, for that matter, that it is pain-free).

It is clear then, that when a woman tells another person that her baby is to be, or was, born by caesarean, this information is likely to be greeted by a multitude of mixed messages: that caesarean birth is the easy way to have a baby, that it is pain-free and risk-free, that it is a dreadful calamity, that it is merely a medical procedure, that it is not really a major operation and that her experience of childbirth is unimportant so long as she and her baby emerge from it alive and well. These are also the messages that we carry with us as pregnancy draws to an end and birth approaches.

3 Born a Cut Above

Caesarean birth itself is both a medical procedure and a profound emotional experience. If you are facing a caesarean or if you have had one and are trying to piece together all that happened to you, it is important to know both medical details about caesareans, and how women actually feel during caesarean childbirth. The way we feel at this time will vary depending on whether the caesarean is carried out as an emergency or whether it is planned in advance, that is elective. Our experience of the birth will also depend on the type of anaesthesia we have.

AN EMERGENCY OR AN ELECTIVE CAESAREAN

Over half of all caesareans are classified as emergency caesareans. The emergency that necessitates the caesarean may arise at any point in the latter half of pregnancy, but it more usually occurs after labour has begun. There are different degrees of emergency. At one end of the spectrum there are the dire emergencies where either the baby's or the mother's life is in danger. At the other end are situations where labour is not progressing well, and although the mother or baby are not distressed, it gradually becomes apparent over the course of hours or days that the labour is unlikely to result in a vaginal birth.

Caesareans that are real emergencies can be very frightening and a woman may be overwhelmed with fear for the safety of her baby. On top of this, most women who have an emergency caesarean are emotionally unprepared for the event and describe feeling a great sense of shock:

It was a matter of 'This baby would be better off out than in' and everything happened so quickly. I was in the operating theatre before I knew what was happening. Trying to put it in perspective, I think it wasn't so much the caesarean, more the emergency that caused the trauma.

Those who have an emergency caesarean after a long and difficult labour describe these feelings of shock too, but also often report a sense of relief when the decision to carry out a caesarean is made:

> When someone mentioned a caesarean as a possibility, it was the light at the end of the tunnel — the only way to finish what I was drowning in the middle of.

Elective caesareans are planned in advance, but the amount of notice women are given varies enormously. Some women know even before they become pregnant that a caesarean will be necessary. Sometimes it will be apparent early in pregnancy that it is on the cards, but in many cases it is only as the end of pregnancy draws near, with just a few weeks or days notice, that the decision to carry out an elective caesarean is made. Elective caesareans are usually carried out before labour begins, typically at around 38 weeks of pregnancy. This has a number of advantages: it will be easier to make arrangements at home, especially if you have other children to look after; if you have decided to have epidural anaesthesia for the birth, you will avoid having to have the epidural set up while you are in labour, when it may be difficult to lie still; in addition you will know who will be carrying out the caesarean and will usually have met them before the operation, which can be very reassuring. You will normally be asked to come into hospital the night before. During this time you will probably have a chance to talk to a midwife or doctor who will explain what will happen, and you may also see the anaesthetist to discuss which type of anaesthetic you would like for the birth.

Sometimes, depending on the reason for the caesarean and on the views of your consultant, it is possible to wait until labour starts spontaneously and for your baby to be delivered by caesarean when you arrive in hospital. Having an elective caesarean after labour has begun also has its advantages. You will know that your baby is ready to be born. You will be able to experience some contractions, something that some women see as an advantage, but others do not! Some women also find waiting until labour starts naturally less clinical and more exciting than having a caesarean on a predetermined date. In addition, the chances of your baby suffering from breathing difficulties at birth are lessened when an elective caesarean is carried out after the onset of labour,[1] and some research suggests that those who have experienced a degree of labour before giving birth by caesarean are more likely to deliver vaginally in subsequent births than those with no previous experience of labour.[2]

There are two situations which fall somewhere between emergency and elective caesareans. The first is when an elective caesarean is planned, but labour begins before the set date, just as this woman describes:

> It was almost an elective caesarean. I was most unwilling to have a doctor decide what my baby's birthday would be, fortunately she solved that problem herself by deciding to arrive the day before! So at least I had the satisfaction of knowing that she was born when she was meant to.

The other situation is when a caesarean is carried out after a trial of labour, when all concerned know that there is a fair chance that a caesarean may be needed. Caesarean mothers who have had a trial of labour are usually emotionally prepared for the possibility of a caesarean delivery and therefore do not experience the same sense of shock that is common after an emergency caesarean. But they may well experience feelings of disappointment, and perhaps wonder what was the point of going through labour. However, many women are pleased to have had a trial of labour, even when it ends in a caesarean, because they know from the evidence of their own body that the caesarean was necessary. Some also feel pleased to have experienced labour:

> I still wonder what it would be like to have a normal delivery, although I did go through a trial of labour and that was fantastic. It has made me feel that at least I had gone through most of what other mums go through except for the actual delivery.

THE ANAESTHETIC DECISION

A caesarean can be carried out under either general or regional anaesthesia. With a general anaesthetic, the woman is unconscious during the birth, whereas with a regional anaesthetic the woman is numbed from the waist downwards (by means of anaesthetic injected into her spine) and remains awake during the caesarean.

There are two main types of regional anaesthesia that are used for caesarean deliveries — epidurals and spinals. In North America, spinals are used more often than epidurals, but in Britain epidurals are far more common than spinals. Of the women who took part in the research for this book who had regional anaesthesia, around 5 out of 6 had an epidural anaesthetic for the caesarean, with only one in 6 having a spinal anaesthetic. The type of regional anaesthetic you are given usually depends on the preferences of your anaesthetist, but it is well worth discussing the issue with him or her if you are particularly keen to have an epidural, or to have a spinal.

There are advantages and disadvantages to both epidurals and spinals. Spinals are faster, sometimes taking as little as ten minutes to set up and take effect, compared with half an hour or more for an epidural. Also, a spinal can sometimes be used when an epidural fails to work properly. Spinals are less likely than epidurals to give incomplete pain relief. In addition, they involve a smaller amount of drugs. These advantages may be offset, however, by a number of disadvantages. Spinal anaesthesia can only be given once, unlike epidurals which can be topped up, and this can be a problem if the operation takes longer than anticipated. One common side-effect of spinals is the 'spinal headache', a severe and debilitating headache than can last for several days, although the incidence of headaches can be reduced to one or 2 per cent by using an extremely fine needle to inject the anaesthetic.[3] Spinal headaches can occur when an epidural anaesthetic is given, but this happens less frequently than with spinal anaesthesia. One final problem with spinals is that they may produce a rapid fall in blood pressure, which can be dangerous. This can also happen with epidurals, but when epidural anaesthesia is used any fall in blood pressure is easier to control and correct. These differences notwithstanding, there are many similarities between epidural and spinal anaesthesia, and what applies to those who have epidural caesareans generally also applies to those who have spinal caesareans. Therefore, for the remainder of this book, I will sometimes simply refer to epidural caesareans rather than caesareans under regional anaesthesia or epidural/spinal caesareans.

Whilst it is the anaesthetist who generally decides between epidural and spinal anaesthesia, it is usually women themselves who make the decision between general and regional anaesthesia. In some cases, however, there is no choice. You will need to have a general anaesthetic if your baby needs to be born very quickly and there is not enough time to administer an epidural, or to top up one that is already in place. Similarly, you may not be able to have an epidural if you have back problems, or if you have low blood pressure, since the further lowering of blood pressure brought about by the epidural could be dangerous. This lowering of the blood pressure can also be dangerous if a woman is already losing blood, so epidural anaesthesia is rarely used when caesareans are carried out for antepartum haemorrhage. You may also be advised to have a general anaesthetic if you have placenta praevia, since caesareans carried out for this reason are sometimes more difficult and may involve greater blood loss. Some anaesthetists would also advise against epidural anaesthetic if you have active herpes because of the small risk of the herpes virus being introduced into the spinal cord. Occasionally, but more rarely, general anaesthesia may be contraindicated, if, for example, a woman has had problems with general anaesthesia in the past.

When we are given a choice of anaesthetic, how do we make this choice? Some women know straight away which type of anaesthetic they prefer, but for others it can be a very difficult decision:

> I think staying awake having a caesarean is a brave thing to do. Well, it took me seven months to decide, and at the last minute I nearly backed out, but I'm glad I didn't.

It is a decision that only you can make. What is the right decision for one woman may not be the right decision for another, but it can help to hear how other women made their decisions.

Over half of all caesarean mothers give birth under general anaesthetic. Sometimes they do so for the medical reasons outlined above, and sometimes they do so out of choice. Although general anaesthesia has some disadvantages, the main one being that you cannot witness the birth of your child, the decision to have a general anaesthetic may well be the right decision for you. None of us should be pressured into having an epidural or feel guilty about opting for general anaesthesia. There are many good reasons for doing so. We may be tired and overwhelmed by labour:

> Even though the epidural worked very well I still chose the general anaesthetic because I wasn't in a fit state to cope with it awake. I was so tired, I just wanted to go to sleep.

If we are in the throes of labour we may not feel able to lie still for the time that it takes administer the epidural:

> I decided to opt for a general anaesthetic because the epidural had been so difficult to set up in my first labour. It was very distressing — how can you lie still, curled up in a ball, when you are in labour and have been for fifteen hours?

We may find the prospect of being awake for an operation very frightening:

> I would very much like to have an epidural if I had to have another caesarean, but at the present time I know I couldn't handle it — I would be too scared.

> The anaesthetist tried to persuade me to have an epidural, but I felt very strongly that if I was going to be cut open I didn't want to be around to see it!

We may find the idea of being awake yet immobilised and helpless very distressing. Or we may fear losing control.

The decision to have a general anaesthetic is sometimes based upon a fear of epidurals. Common fears are that the epidural will be very painful to set up, and that it may damage us or even lead to paralysis. Whilst a minority of women do find the setting up of an epidural painful, this is not usually the case, since a local injection is given before the epidural needle is inserted into the spine. Occasionally women experience numbness or weakness in the legs or backache after an epidural but this is invariably temporary.[4] The risk of paralysis is negligible. The few cases when epidural anaesthesia have led to paralysis all occurred over twenty years ago and were the result of either the wrong drug being injected into the spine, or infection prior to the use of adequate aseptic procedures. Nowadays the type of drug used is checked by two people, and great care is taken to prevent infection.

Sometimes the attitudes of medical staff influence the type of anaesthetic a woman chooses. Whilst epidural caesareans are encouraged in most hospitals nowadays, this is not always so:

> Even the female staff could not understand why I wanted to be awake for the caesarean. One said, 'Go to sleep, dear, and get it all over with.' Another said, 'You don't want to be awake, dear, it's not very nice.'

The fact that partners are rarely allowed to be present at a caesarean under general anaesthetic, but are usually encouraged to be present at an epidural caesarean, can also influence anaesthetic decisions. Sometimes women choose to have a general anaesthetic for this reason:

> We both wanted my husband to be present for the birth if it was a normal delivery, but my husband didn't want to witness the caesarean and I didn't think it was fair to expect him to do so. This was mainly the reason why I chose the general anaesthetic as I couldn't face the operation alone.

In other cases, women decide on epidural anaesthesia for the very fact that their partners can be present at the birth.

The main reason, however, for opting for an epidural is so that the mother herself can see her baby being born and welcome the child into the world. Other reasons for choosing to have this type of anaesthetic include the facts that women are less likely to feel groggy after an epidural than a general anaesthetic; that it carries less risk to the mother; and that smaller amounts of anaesthetic drugs reach the baby during the caesarean.

Another reason for choosing an epidural is the fear of general anaesthetic failure. Although such failures are rare, many women have become very aware of this problem as a result of the widespread publicity surrounding recent court cases brought by women who have suffered in this way:

> The thing I'm most scared of is the anaesthetic, being awake and feeling it all but not being able to tell anyone. I'm not scared of feeling anything with an epidural because I would be able to tell someone.

In addition to general and regional anaesthesia, there have been some reported cases of women having caesareans using acupuncture, being awake and in no pain. Rarer still are cases where caesareans have been carried out under hypnosis. These types of anaesthesia are, however, very unusual and will not be on offer under normal circumstances.

WHAT HAPPENS

Here I will be describing the procedures that need to be carried out in preparation for a caesarean, the administration of the anaesthetic and the operation itself. Some women find it helpful to know what happens during the operation, but others do not. If you would prefer not to know the details of the operation, then skip the relevant section.

There are many procedures that are necessary before a caesarean can begin. The order in which these are carried out will vary from hospital to hospital, with the type of anaesthetic used and whether it is an emergency or elective caesarean. Whether they are carried out in the delivery room, in a side room or in the operating theatre, and before or after the anaesthetic is administered, also varies depending on the situation.

You will invariably be asked to sign a consent form to show that you agree to the caesarean being carried out. The top part of your pubic hair will be shaved, and an intravenous drip will be put into your hand. A catheter (a fine plastic or rubber tube) will be inserted to empty your bladder. This is sometimes uncomfortable, but should not be painful. If you are wearing make-up or nail varnish these will be removed so that the anaesthetist can observe any changes in the colour of your lips and nails during the operation. You will also be asked to remove contact lenses and to take off any jewellery, apart from your wedding ring which will be taped to your finger. A paper cap will be put over your hair. A blood pressure cuff will then be placed on your arm so that your blood pressure can be monitored during the caesarean, and adhesive discs will be attached to your chest to pick up your heart rate. A diathermy plate, which is part of the equipment used to control bleeding during the operation, may be strapped around your leg. You will be asked to drink antacid solution to neutralise any acid in your stomach. Just before the operation begins you will be asked to breathe in some oxygen through a mask for the benefit of the baby.

You will need to discuss the choice of anaesthetic with your anaesthetist, who will also ask you questions about your medical history. If you are having regional anaesthesia this will need to be set up, unless you already have an epidural in place, in which case it will be topped up. To administer a regional anaesthetic, you will be asked to lie on your left side and to curl up into a ball, or alternatively to sit on the side of the bed, with your feet on a stool and your elbows resting on your knees. A small area of your back will be painted with antiseptic solution. You will then be given an injection of local anaesthetic to numb the area of your spine where the epidural or spinal needle is to be inserted. Next, the anaesthetist will insert a needle between the vertibrae of the lower part of your spine. If you are having an epidural the needle will go in as far as the space just outside the dura, which is the sheath of membrane that protects the spinal cord. A fine plastic tube is then threaded down the needle, which may cause you to feel a sharp, momentary twinge down one leg, and the needle is taken out. The tube is then taped to your back to hold it in place, and the anaesthetic is injected down the tube.

If you are having a spinal anaesthetic, the needle will be inserted between the vertebrae of your spine, but instead of stopping short of the dura it penetrates the dura and enters the centremost part of the spinal column which contains cerebrospinal fluid. The anaesthetic is then injected directly into this fluid, and the needle is removed. You are then rolled gently from side to side to help disperse the anaesthetic.

Epidurals generally take between ten and twenty minutes to set up and another fifteen or twenty minutes to take effect, whereas spinals take less time. Gradually you will feel you legs and abdomen go numb and loose sensation. You may still be able to move your toes — this does not mean the epidural is not working properly. You may feel dizzy, shaky or nauseous for a while as the epidural takes effect. This is due to a temporary drop in blood pressure caused by the epidural. Finally, the anaesthetist will check that the epidural has taken effect either by pricking your abdomen with a sharp needle or by using a cold spray.

If you are having general anaesthesia, an anaesthetic drug will be injected into your intravenous drip and within around thirty seconds you will be asleep. As this takes effect, the anaesthetist will press firmly on your neck to prevent vomiting. Some women are aware of this pressure on the neck, others are not. The anaesthetist then administers another injection to relax all your muscles, and passes a tube down your throat into your trachea (windpipe). This tube is connected to a ventilator machine which breathes for you during the operation and administers a mixture of gases to ensure that you remain unconscious. The siting of this tube also prevents the inhalation of the stomach's contents, which can be very dangerous.

Now that you are anaesthetised the operation can begin. You will be lying on an operating table that is slightly tilted to the left. Your abdomen will be painted with an antiseptic solution and you will be draped in sterile cloths, leaving your lower abdomen exposed. If you are under regional anaesthetic, the cloths will be draped over a bar above your chest so that you cannot see the operation itself, although you may see it reflected in the large circular lights above the operating table.

The obstetrician begins by making a cut along the skin that is 4–7″ long. Nowadays, this cut is nearly always a horizontal one, just below the pubic hairline. This type of cut is known as a lower segment or transverse incision, a bikini cut or a Pfannenstiel incision. However, in around 2 per cent of caesareans a vertical or classical incision, also known as a midline or para-median cut, is made, running from around the top of your pubic hairline to just below your navel. A classical incision may be necessary in dire emergencies, since classical caesareans take slightly less time to perform. If your baby is lying in a transverse position a classical incision will usually be carried out because it is difficult to get a transverse baby out through a lower segment incision. Triplets are also often delivered through a classical incision. There is a growing trend for the use of classical incisions when premature babies are delivered by caesarean, but there has been some debate about this, and the practice has yet to be fully evaluated.[5] A classical incision is also sometimes necessary if you have already had two or three lower segment caesareans. Occasionally the incision that you can see on your abdomen is different from the one on your uterus.

After this initial incision, the obstetrician then cuts through the fatty tissue just below your skin and the sheath that covers your abdominal muscles. A small cut is made between the muscles and they are gently separated to reveal a thin membrane known as the peritoneum. This membrane surrounds the abdominal organs, including the bladder and the uterus. The bladder is carefully eased away from the front of the uterus, and an incision is made in the uterus itself. Next the membranes are broken and the amniotic fluid that surrounds the baby throughout pregnancy is suctioned out.

Your baby can now be born. The obstetrician reaches into your uterus, while the assisting doctor presses down firmly two or three times on your abdomen over the top part of the uterus to help ease the baby out. If you have regional anaesthesia you may well be asked to bear down at this point to help push your baby out. Forceps are sometimes used to deliver the baby's head. It takes around five to ten minutes from the start of the operation until the baby is born. As your newborn enters the world his cord will be clamped and cut, and any mucus will be suctioned out of his nose and mouth. The paediatrician will then check that he is breathing well and assess his condition. If you have had regional anaesthesia, your baby will now be placed in your arms. If you are under general anaesthetic the baby will normally be given to your partner to greet and cuddle, only minutes after the birth.

Next, the placenta and membranes are removed and the placenta is checked. Then the sewing up begins, which generally takes between thirty minutes and an hour. The uterus is repaired and the abdomen is stitched back in layers. The internal stitches are made with dissolvable thread. The final layer of skin is closed with dissolvable stitches, clips or non-dissolving stitches (either a number of stitches or one running stitch secured with beads at the ends) that will be removed during your hospital stay. Sometimes, a small plastic tube, known as a drain, may be put into the wound to drain away any blood that might collect there. The wound is then covered with a dressing, and the operation is over.

If you have had a general anaesthetic, you will be given an antidote to reverse the effects of the muscle relaxant, the anaesthetic gases will be turned off and the tracheal tube will be removed. When you come round you may find that you are still in the operating theatre, or you may be in a side room. In normal circumstances, your partner and baby will be with you as you wake up, or they will arrive soon afterwards. You may even wake to find your baby in bed with you.

HOW IT FEELS

So far I have described what actually happens during a caesarean birth, but this tells us little about what it actually feels like to give birth in this way. I have collected together comments from a number of caesarean mothers to illustrate women's positive and negative experiences of caesarean birth under both general and regional anaesthesia.

Our feelings when we have a caesarean with general anaesthesia are many and varied. For some, it is a very positive experience. Indeed, around a third of women who have a general anaesthetic for one caesarean say they would choose this type of anaesthetic again in future caesarean births:[6]

> When I was told that I would have to have a caesarean I just remember thinking at least I wouldn't have any more contractions. I wasn't upset that I couldn't give birth naturally and now nine months later it still hasn't upset me.

Everyone was extremely kind, explaining exactly what would happen and how I would feel. The anaesthetist introduced herself and explained her role and what I would see and feel in theatre. We found everyone was very reassuring.

I lay awake for a while in the theatre whilst they waited for the doctor. But at least all the time I felt included and was told what was going on all the time.

There was an air of excitement in the room from the moment the caesarean was decided upon, as we knew then it would not be long now and we'd have the baby.

Luckily a nurse had taken our camera into theatre and took some marvellous photos of Daniel having just been born, being checked by the paediatrician and weighed, etc., which are lovely to look back on.

I was told I had a daughter and then my husband passed her to me. The midwife helped me to hold her — I was elated, overjoyed. All I could think about was how beautiful my baby was. I didn't care how she'd been born, or think about the cut across my tummy.

I came round from the anaesthetic and felt great. I was very sore afterwards, there is no getting away from that, but it just doesn't seem to matter when you gaze at this wonderful human being you have created. I held her while I was being wheeled onto the ward and I bonded instantly. I couldn't wait to breastfeed.

For some women, caesarean childbirth under general anaesthesia is not such a positive experience. What follows are comments describing very difficult experiences of caesarean birth with general anaesthesia. It is important to remember, however, that the experiences of the majority of women fall somewhere between the two extremes presented here:

It was horrendous. Emotionally I was not prepared for it. I was terrified of being unconscious, of waking up, of not waking up.

The consultant was ages coming to the theatre. I was lying on the table, lights everywhere, all the theatre staff gowned up, waiting for this man. I was so petrified I could hardly breathe. I should have been in Sainsbury's or watching the news and here I was in this nightmare.

I remember looking at everything and wondering if I would ever be a part of life again.

I was very scared before the caesarean. I shook so much that they had to hold me on the operating table. I hated the oxygen mask being forced on my face; everyone dashing about sticking monitors on my chest; the anaesthetist trying to find my vein — it seemed like hours instead of minutes.

A doctor proceeded to put the anaesthetic into my arm, at the same time a second doctor held a mask over my face and a third squeezed my throat. I literally felt as though I would not wake up again. When I woke up nobody came to tell me what I'd had. I was facing the other way and as no one realised I was awake, I could overhear a nurse saying how 'he sounded hungry', it was like I didn't exist.

After the birth, I remember waking up in excruciating pain. I was still in the theatre, with all these masked faces around me. I was still very drowsy and everything was hazy. All I could think of was the immense pain I was feeling at that moment — not even of the baby. I remember being wheeled to the ward and my husband standing over me. I remember asking him what the baby was, and if it was all right. He said we had a daughter and that she was fine. He told me later that I had asked him this at least a dozen times. I do not remember.

Next, I was wheeled into a side room. I don't remember feeling happy or anything, just relieved it was over and conscious of a terrible, terrible pain at the bottom of my abdomen.

Women also vary enormously in how they feel during epidural caesareans. In my research, a quarter of women reported feeling happy during caesareans with regional anaesthesia, the majority said they felt both happy and frightened, and a small minority were just plain frightened.[7] Those whose experience was primarily positive described it as follows:

I had an epidural which took a lot of setting up, but the staff were really good, reassuring me all the time.

I felt intrigued by the new sensation, thrilled by what I perceived as a trial on my self-control.

The actual operation was really good, I didn't even know they had started. Everyone kept asking me if I was OK and it was really cheerful in there! The operation took less than ten minutes and we were given the baby straight away. I'd have another caesarean without even thinking twice.

I can describe the sensation of the surgery as similar to the strong movements of the baby during the months he lived in my womb — so it certainly wasn't painful.

The birth was a wonderful experience. I felt no pain. I was only aware of a slight tugging and pulling.

Being asked to bear down to help deliver my child was wonderful. To be positively involved despite the elective caesar was an unexpected bonus.

To me it was a fantastic experience. I wanted to know everything that was going on. I can honestly say I found it enjoyable and the whole team of doctors, anaesthetists, nurses, midwives, etc., were all really brilliant.

It was the most beautiful experience to watch as my baby daughter was lifted up above the curtain in front of my waist. She looked so perfect, and of course I was so anaesthetised I felt no pain. Everything appeared in slow motion and it was all worth while.

Slowly he opened his eyes, moved his lips gently and had his first suckle. I was so excited I forgot to sleep until the following morning.

It was just like a 'real' birth and not an operation at all.

The sewing-up stage of the caesarean seemed very quick.

I was high for months afterwards. I still get elated thinking about it. It was so easy, so painless.

Unfortunately not everyone feels like this during epidural caesareans. Being awake during surgery is not always easy. Indeed, according to one survey around a third of women felt ill at ease during the delivery, both physically and psychologically.[8] Nevertheless, for the majority of caesarean mothers, the joy of seeing their newborn enter the world seems to offset any fear or distress during the operation since the vast majority would opt for regional anaesthesia in future caesareans.[9] But the following comments serve to remind us that epidural caesareans can be very distressing, and that this type of anaesthesia is not right for everyone:

It was like having a tooth out. I knew exactly what time the birth would be and had plenty of time to worry about it the night before.

I was so frightened that I couldn't stop shaking.

After thirty minutes the anaesthetist still had not managed to insert the needle and I was getting very upset (my husband passed out!).

While I was given the epidural I felt like a lamb led to the slaughter. It was such an invasive action and certainly not painless! The sensation of feeling my legs 'disappear' was very worrying, and I felt utterly helpless being paralysed from the waist down.

When I looked up, the theatre light acted like a magnifying mirror, something I hadn't been warned about, there seemed to be gallons of blood, and I started to feel very sick and shaky.

The whole time I remember being absolutely terrified, and I mean really terrified. The surgeon said, 'Are we all ready?' My first thoughts were, 'I've changed my mind, I don't really want this baby! After a struggle Alex was pulled out of my stomach, that was an awful feeling. It felt like they were pulling a snail out of its shell.

I wasn't prepared for the noise of the cutting. It sounded like scissors on a thick fabric. I wish someone had warned me.

I could feel the pushing and pulling as they got the baby out (unpleasant but not painful). I was being sick when the baby was born.

I spent most of the time with my eyes tightly closed, wishing it was all over. But it seemed to go on and on and on. At one point I thought I was dying. Because of my shaking, the blood pressure and heart monitors kept falling off and making that high-pitched bleep that you get on TV when people are dead.

I just wanted to be anywhere but on that table.

ANAESTHETIC FAILURE

I found the topic of anaesthetic failure a difficult one to broach, for it is a nightmarish situation that none of us wish to contemplate. But although anaesthetic failure is rare, it does sometimes occur, and this book would not be complete without giving some consideration to this issue.

It is estimated that in around one in every 100 operations under general anaesthetic the patient has some awareness during the operation.[10] But in most instances, it is merely a case of hearing snatches of conversation. However, in one in every 2,500 operations the patient experiences pain during the operation.[11]

This is slightly more likely to occur in caesareans than in other types of operation because anaesthetic levels are kept low in the mistaken belief that larger doses might harm the baby.[12] In 1988, Margaret Ackers was the first caesarean mother who suffered anaesthetic failure to take her case to court, and she succeeded in winning compensation and, most importantly, public acknowledgement of what had happened to her. Since then a number of other women have followed her lead, and the resulting publicity given to these cases means that the public has become aware of what has been described as 'one of medicine's better kept secrets'.[13]

When general anesthesia fails the patient feels part or all of the operation, but is unable to move or speak because of the muscle relaxant drug that is administered when general anaesthesia is used. This experience is profoundly distressing, and is often described as like being buried alive. The severity of the trauma has been likened to that suffered by those involved in aircraft disasters or by torture victims.[14] Added to this is the further trauma of not being believed, of being told by medical staff or family and friends that it must have been a dream or in the imagination. On a more positive note, the widespread publicity that resulted from the court cases means that women who suffer in this way are now more likely to be believed. It also means that anaesthetists are now looking very closely at the problem of anaesthetic awareness and are considering ways of minimising or eliminating this risk, so that in future anaesthetic failure may become an even rarer occurrence.

Little publicity has been given to the fact that regional anaesthesia can also fail. Such failure is, in fact, more common than general anaesthetic failure, although in some ways it is not quite as traumatic since the woman can tell the anaesthetist that she is in pain and measures can be taken to alleviate it.

In around 5 per cent of epidurals the anaesthetic fails to work, and in a further 5 per cent it works on one side only.[15] In the majority of these cases, however, the fact that the epidural is not working becomes apparent before the caesarean begins, allowing a different form of anaesthesia to be used. One problem that is not usually apparent before the caesarean is underway is that epidural anaesthesia can sometimes be patchy, with areas called 'windows' being unaffected by the anaesthesia.[16] An additional problem is that the ovaries, the fallopian tubes and parts of the uterus have a nerve supply that may not be completely blocked by the epidural, and women occasionally report pain when these organs are handled.[17]

Sometimes, if pain is mild or temporary, women are able to cope with it by using breathing techniques, but this can still be a very distressing experience:

> Unfortunately the epidural did not work fully and so I had to put all my concentration onto bearing the pain to avoid a general anaesthetic. This made me not really appreciate the arrival of my baby. I could not believe the pain, it was something I could never describe. I can remember thinking I deserved it, as I would have had pain in a normal delivery. My husband had taken some photos of the actual caesarean, and I could not look at these until two months later.

Sometimes, when pain is experienced during an epidural caesarean, women are given entonox (a mixture of gas and oxygen which helps to relieve pain) to breathe or intravenous painkillers. However, a general anaesthetic will often be necessary. This woman wrote:

> I was given the epidural with no problem. During the operation before the babies were taken out, I began to feel unbearable pain. I started using breathing techniques through an eternity of agony. I remember being told the babies were boys and saying to the anaesthetist that I was in absolute agony. From then on everything went blank.

The way caesarean birth is experienced depends not just on factors such as whether it was an emergency or an elective caesarean, the type of anaesthesia used or on how well the anaesthesia works, but also on the less tangible factors discussed in Chapter 2, such as our expectations of vaginal and caesarean birth and the amount of information and preparation we have received. There are three other very important psychological factors that play a large part in determining how we experience caesarean childbirth. These are whether or not we perceive the caesarean to be entirely necessary; how involved and informed we are in decisions about labour and delivery; and the extent to which we feel cared for and supported by the medical professionals looking after us.

PERCEPTIONS OF NECESSITY

Women who do not feel that their caesareans were essential to ensure the health and safety of themselves or their babies, or those who believe that a caesarean could and should have been avoided, are more likely to report having difficult feelings about the birth.[18] The importance of perceptions of necessity is also apparent in the fact that many caesarean mothers describe the main thing that made them feel positive about having a caesarean as being the knowledge that it was essential to save their baby's life, or to avoid the baby becoming seriously handicapped.

There are a number of situations that can leave a woman feeling that her caesarean was not absolutely necessary. Occasionally, clearcut mistakes or misdiagnoses occur. But more common than this are the 'grey areas' where medical opinions differ about whether or not a caesarean is necessary, such as with breech birth, prolonged labour, mild fetal distress and repeat caesareans. One caesarean mother said:

> The caesarean was especially difficult to cope with as I was told it was my consultant's 'policy' to give all first-time mothers whose babies were breech presentation a caesarean delivery. I am always suspicious of blanket policies which do not take into account individual circumstances.

> I was told that I wouldn't automatically be given another caesarean. The situation would be assessed at 37 weeks. When decision time came I was really hoping for a vaginal delivery, but the consultant walked into the room, straight past me, read my notes and said he thought he'd go for a caesarean the same as last time. I did protest, but he said it would be safer, so I agreed, but I was very disappointed. I certainly don't feel I was given the chance of a vaginal delivery.

Occasionally caesareans are thought to have been carried out for non-medical reasons such as for the convenience of the obstetrician:

> During one examination I was told by the obstetrician that he thought I was going to deliver the baby by myself. On the next examination he decided, in his own words, 'No change, repeat section, enough is enough, OK.' I was so upset and very confused. I was very depressed for the first few days and cried almost constantly. My husband later told me that after my son was delivered the obstetrician gave him the news that he had had a son, then said, 'Oh well, I can go home now.' My husband felt that the section was done for his convenience and was also very upset and angry.

Many women also report doubts about the necessity of their caesareans when they have been subjected to an escalation of routine interventions during labour which has led to fetal or maternal distress, necessitating a caesarean. The caesarean is typically perceived as having been necessary in the prevailing circumstances, but nevertheless as a caesarean that could possibly have been avoided:

> Although I thought I had come to terms with having a caesarean, somewhere part of me remains convinced that I would have birthed my daughter normally and safely if I had been given the time and support from the hospital.

Even when caesareans are carried out for clearcut medical reasons, these reasons may not have been fully explained to the woman concerned. In fact, almost half of the women in my research felt that they had not had an adequate explanation for their caesareans by the time they left hospital.[19] This may well have left them wondering if their caesareans were really necessary.

THE IMPORTANCE OF BEING INVOLVED AND INFORMED

Whether a woman and her partner participate in and feel involved in the decision to carry out a caesarean and in the events that lead up to it also has an important influence on the way caesarean childbirth is experienced. Those who feel involved and informed tend to view their caesareans more positively:[20]

> It can still be your birth, despite any amount of technology. It was so in our case. I had written a birth plan, almost every point of which had to be rejected. But the staff did refer to it, point by point, throughout labour, always explaining, asking and leaving the decision up to me and to my husband when I had gone beyond consultation.

A birth plan is a written statement summarising your wishes for the birth. Writing one is a way of letting those caring for you during the birth of your baby know your preferences. Birth plans are not irrevocable, they can be, and often are, modified in the light of experiences during labour and of problems that may arise. When used appropriately, these plans can encourage discussion and parental involvement in childbearing decisions. Many women who have made birth plans and have had caesareans, either emergency or elective, found them beneficial. Nevertheless, a small number of caesarean mothers stated that not making a birth plan was something that helped them to feel positive about their birth experience, since they felt this enabled them to keep an open mind about the birth, without setting up hopes and expectations that were not to be fulfilled. But most of us will inevitably have hopes and expectations about a forthcoming birth, whether we write them down or not. If you decide to write a birth plan you might want to include some of the ideas on caesarean prevention and on helping yourself to a better caesarean that are discussed in Chapter 10. It is a good idea to discuss the points you include in your birth plan with your midwife or doctor in advance.

Sheila Kitzinger introduced the concept of 'autonomous birth' to describe birth experiences like the one cited above, in which women have the opportunity to consider the advantages and disadvantages of different alternatives and come to their own decisions.[21] When caesarean birth is conducted in this way, it can be a very positive and empowering experience.

The concept of informed consent is also important here. No

medical procedure, including interventions during labour and caesarean deliveries, should be carried out without your consent. To do so may well constitute an assault.[22] However, medical procedures are sometimes carried out without consent, and this often leaves women feeling disempowered and out of control:

> A student doctor finally broke my waters after three attempts. I was put on a drip and on two monitors. Everything was done without consulting me. I felt as though they took over. I was not in control at all.

In the USA, there have been a number of court-ordered caesareans, where obstetricians have taken out court orders to force women to undergo caesarean sections.[23] There have not, as yet, been any such cases in Britain, but the experiences of many women indicate that caesareans are sometimes carried out without full, informed consent:

> After another examination a doctor muttered under his breathe, 'Section.' My husband only just heard what he said and I didn't quite catch it. While the midwife went out to get the operation preparation trolley my husband told me what had been said. Nothing was explained to me. One of the worst things about having a section for me was decisions being made over my head without any regard for my thoughts or feelings.

Despite the fact that Murray Enkin and his colleagues include 'Failing to involve women in decisions about their care' in their list of obstetric practices that should be abandoned in the light of the available evidence,[24] there are still too many doctors like obstetrician Elliot Philipp who believes that 'when something abnormal arises, no matter how well one explains the situation, women, even women doctors, find it hard to make decisions about the way to conduct their own labours'.[25] While such views prevail, some women will continue to have childbearing decisions taken out of their hands, and to suffer the negative psychological consequences that this can bring about.

CARE AND SUPPORT DURING CHILDBIRTH

The final factor that influences the way we experience caesarean birth is the amount of care and support we receive at this time. Such support has a large effect on our subsequent feelings about the caesarean.[26] When a caesarean is carried out after labour, the support given during labour can be crucial:

> The delivery staff, doctors and specialists, were really marvellous and supportive. I think they were more disappointed than I was that I would need an operation.

When such care and support is lacking, this can have deep and long-lasting effects:

> The midwives just sat and watched me and did nothing and I felt debased.

A supportive and caring atmosphere is also very important during the difficult time just before the caesarean is carried out:

> I did not enjoy the pre-surgery gossip in the theatre. It was like standing on the edge of a party and no one knowing you were there even though the party is being given in your honour!

The difference that support can make is well illustrated in the following account by a woman whose first baby was born by elective caesarean under general anaesthetic, and whose second child was born by emergency caesarean after a failed induction, this time under epidural anaesthesia. Although the experiences differed in the type of anaesthetic used and in whether the caesarean was emergency or elective, what really made the difference between the two experiences was the attitude and supportiveness of the staff:

> When I had my first caesarean I remember asking the staff questions, but their answers were superficial, and never reassured me. I was last on the operating list and as it was

lunchtime when they wheeled me down, it seemed to me they just wanted to get the operation over with as soon as possible and get off to have their dinner. It may have been 'just another section' to them, but it certainly wasn't for me! The staff were milling around me, putting on electrodes, shoving needles in with no explanation. From the other end of the room the anaesthetist fired only partially audible questions at me, not even waiting for an answer, but still wrote something down. He hadn't even bothered to visit me prior to the op which I thought was unusual. I felt like a lump of meat . . . When my second daughter was born it was so different. This time the staff were brilliant. They sat for ages listening to me, answering my questions and explaining in detail any of my queries. One midwife even went through her epidural section with me, saying it was the best day of her life. The anaesthetist visited me and explained the epidural to me at great length to help reassure me. The whole attitude of the staff there was so totally different. They were so genuinely friendly and caring and I was put so much more at ease than last time.

The amount of support we receive during our stay in hospital also appears to play an important role in determining how we feel about our caesarean birth experience.[27] It is to the hospital stay and the early days following a caesarean that we now turn.

4 Early Days

THE HOSPITAL STAY

The way we feel during our stay in hospital varies enormously from woman to woman. For some it is a restful time which lays the foundation for speedy physical and emotional recovery. For others it is an exhausting and distressing time — the hospital stay is sometimes described as the worst part of having a caesarean. What is often of crucial importance in determining how we feel at this time is the amount of care and support we receive during our stay.

For the women in my research there was a strong association between amount of support received during the hospital stay and subsequent feelings about the caesarean.[1] Those who felt that they did not receive enough support at this time were also more likely to be depressed after the birth and to report having problems in forming a relationship with their baby.[2] This concept of support includes: practical help with activities such as getting in and out of bed, walking and washing; support during medical procedures, for example when stitches are taken out; assisting the mother in caring for her new baby; help with breastfeeding; and emotional support — listening, answering questions, explaining the reasons for the caesarean, and talking through the birth experience.

Unfortunately, we do not always receive the sort of care and support we need during our stay in hospital, due to cutbacks and staff shortages. In 1988, nearly one fifth of midwifery posts in Britain remained unfilled, with greater shortfalls in some areas of the country.[3] It is caesarean mothers, with our longer stay in hospital and our increased needs as post-operative patients, who often feel the effects of these staff shortages most keenly.[4]

The hospital stay begins in the recovery room, when you and

your partner are usually able to spend some time alone with your newborn, welcoming her and getting to know her. Some women report feeling very groggy at this time, particularly after a general anaesthetic, but others feel alert and well. After a while you will be transferred to the maternity ward, where you will normally stay for the next five to ten days.

You may be given a single room or you may be put in a shared ward, which could contain anything from two to twenty new mothers and babies. In my research, around a quarter of caesarean mothers had a single room for the whole of their stay, around a third spent their entire stay in a shared ward and the remainder initially had single rooms and later transferred to a shared ward. There are both advantages and disadvantages to being in a single room. Some women value the privacy that it provides:

> I feel having a single room for the first few days certainly helped as I felt such a horrendous wreck. I could be alone with my husband to sort out my feelings in private.

Some women report feeling isolated and forgotten in single rooms. Perhaps the main drawback to being in a shared ward is the lack of sleep:[5]

> I hardly got any sleep, that was the worst thing about being in hospital. When my baby was quiet it was someone else's baby crying.

Nevertheless, this disadvantage is sometimes outweighed by the advantage of having the company of other mothers:

> The sharing of all our problems helped enormously, as nothing seems as bad when you can talk about it.

If you are in a shared ward and would prefer a single room or vice versa, it is sometimes possible to change, so it is worthwhile asking.

Initially, you will have a drip in your hand and a catheter in place. You may also have a drain (a thin piece of tubing draining away any blood and fluid that collects in your caesarean wound).

How long these stay in place varies between hospitals, but drips are usually removed after twelve to forty-eight hours, the catheter is typically taken out within twenty-four hours and, in general, drains are removed after one or two days.

The dressing on your wound may be removed after a couple of days, or may remain in place until your stitches are taken out. Stitches (or clips) tend to be removed around five days after the birth, although they will be left in place a few days longer if you have a classical (vertical) scar. Having stitches out is sometimes uncomfortable but it is not usually painful. Your scar will probably feel more comfortable and less taut once the stitches have been removed.

Your temperature, pulse and blood pressure will be checked regularly during your stay. Your abdomen will also be checked to ensure that your uterus is returning to its normal size. You may well notice that your abdomen is somewhat distended, due to wind accumulating in the bowels. This is common after a caesarean, but is only a temporary effect. Like any newly delivered mother, you will have a discharge, known as lochia, which is similar to a period. This may last for up to six weeks, but the amount of lochia tends to be minimal after the first couple of weeks. It is often more comfortable after a caesarean to wear large knickers that come up to your waist since these are less likely to irritate your scar.

In most hospitals you will be encouraged to get out of bed within twenty-four hours of the birth. Walking after a caesarean is painful, but it is important as it improves your circulation and helps to prevent thrombosis (blood clots in the legs). For the same reason, it is a good idea to wriggle your toes and circle your ankles in bed right from the start. You will need assistance in getting out of bed and will be helped to walk to a chair by your bed or to the toilet. It is important to try to walk as upright as possible and to avoid the 'caesarean shuffle'. Although walking is difficult at first, it does become a lot easier after a few days. Slip-on slippers are useful, since bending over to pull them on is not easy.

You will not be given anything to eat whilst your drip is in place, although you may be encouraged to have sips of water. You are unlikely to be hungry or thirsty as you will receive fluid and nutrition through the drip. After this you will be offered either a light diet, such as soup and ice cream, or the ordinary hospital diet. Initially you will have meals in bed, but after a few days you will be expected to take them in the dining room. It is often helpful if your partner brings in some snacks such as fruit or cereal as well.

Once your catheter has been removed you will need to go to the toilet. In some hospitals catheters are removed very early on and a bedpan is used, but more often you will be helped to walk to the toilet. Passing urine is not usually painful. You are unlikely to have a bowel movement during the first few days after a caesarean since the operation tends to make your system somewhat sluggish — you may be offered a laxative, suppository or enema to help. Opening your bowels for the first time can be very uncomfortable, but it helps if you support your scar with your hands and try to relax.

You will be able to have a wash as soon as you are able to walk to the bathroom. It is also useful to keep a supply of wet wipes by your bed so that you can freshen up whenever you feel like it. After a few days you may have a bath or shower — hospitals vary in which they recommend. If you have a bath you will need some assistance at first since it is not easy to get in and out of the bath after a caesarean. You may also need help if you take a shower:

> When I went in the shower on my third day I had to drip dry, then I dropped my pants on the floor. I couldn't pick them up and I had to pull the emergency cord for some help. I laugh about it now, but at the time I was so embarrassed.

Rest and sleep are very important after a caesarean, but are not always easy to come by in a busy hospital with a new baby to care for. In fact, more than half of the women in my research said they did not get enough sleep during their hospital stay, with some getting as little as two or three hours a night. You may be offered sleeping tablets if you are very tired and unable to sleep.

There are many reasons why caesarean mothers find it difficult to sleep. After a general anaesthetic you will need to sleep in a propped-up position for the first few nights to help clear your chest and lungs, and some women find it difficult to sleep like this. If you are in a shared ward, you may also find it hard to sleep because of the noise of babies crying or other ward noises. Your own baby may be fractious and keep you awake. If your baby has been taken into the nursery at night, you may lie awake wondering if she is all right:

> At night I lay in bed unable to move, hot, uncomfortable, dead tired but unable to sleep. Max was in the nursery and I could hear babies yelling, I kept thinking it was him and how he should be with me, but I was too weak to care for him. I just lay there and cried, I felt so miserable.

Often we are unable to sleep because the whole experience — labour, the caesarean, having a new baby — is going round and round in our head as we try to make some sense of all that has happened to us. Another reason why we may have difficulty in sleeping is post-operative pain.

COPING WITH PAIN

The amount of pain experienced after a caesarean varies enormously. Some women experience very little:

> After the initial pain I suffered little discomfort and was walking about far easier than mothers with episiotomies.

> After my first section I took (and did not need) no painkillers at all. The second time around I found that I needed some every night before going to bed. I found Paracetomol perfectly adequate.

However, research indicates that up to 75 per cent of patients suffer from moderate to severe pain after abdominal surgery,[6] and the majority of caesarean mothers experience some degree of pain. For some women the post-operative pain is the most difficult aspect of caesarean birth:

> Once the epidural wore off, I was in pain every time I moved, even though I asked for and received four hourly analgesics.

My stomach felt very bruised, the epidural site on my back was sore, my arm hurt where the drip had been sited and I had sore and painful nipples.

My first feeling was absolute shock that anything could be so painful. I suppose I had vaguely thought that caesareans were a less painful form of childbirth. It hurt me to cough, laugh or even move slightly. Everything seemed a dreadful effort, I felt totally incapacitated.

It is unclear why some people suffer more post-operative pain than others, but it is a fact that the amount of pain experienced by patients undergoing the same operation can vary tenfold.[7] If you do experience more pain than other caesarean mothers, it is important that you do not see this as a reflection of some weakness on your part. The degree of pain you experience will depend not only on your own pain threshold but also on a number of other factors, such as the type of anaesthesia you had — women generally experience less pain after a caesarean with regional anaesthesia because in this situation a more gentle operating technique is required. Post-operative pain can also vary depending on whether the caesarean was carried out before the onset of labour, early in labour or after a long labour. It is not uncommon for women who have had more than one caesarean to report large differences in the amount of pain experienced after each birth.

The caesarean wound itself is not the only source of pain. Many caesarean mothers suffer from wind pains which can be quite severe. Peppermint water, fennel tea and charcoal biscuits can be helpful in alleviating wind. Some women also suffer from afterpains as the uterus contracts to return to its normal size during the first week or so after birth, something that can be painful for both vaginally-delivered and caesarean mothers. You may find that your breasts feel quite uncomfortable when your milk comes in. In addition, if you have had general anaesthesia, you might find that you have a sore throat due to the siting of tracheal tube.

You will be offered pain relief to help alleviate pain. Initially, this will be in the form of injections of painkillers such as

Omnopon or pethidine. Although traces of these drugs will be present in your breastmilk, the amount involved is very small and will not harm your baby. In a small but increasing number of hospitals, post-operative patients are given what is known as patient-controlled analgesia in which the patient herself presses a button at her side whenever she feels pain returning and a small dose of pain medication is automatically released into her bloodstream. If your caesarean was carried out with epidural anaesthesia, the epidural catheter may be left in place and the epidural topped up to provide pain relief in the first twenty-four hours. After a day or so, you may be offered painkilling tablets instead of injections, and after a few more days Paracetomol tablets are usually all that is needed. Such tablets will not harm your baby if you are breastfeeding. Whilst most of us find pain relief both necessary and helpful, it is important to remember that you are not obliged to accept what is on offer — some women experience very little pain and do not need pain relief, and others prefer to manage without. Similarly, if you are in a lot of pain you should certainly ask whether it is possible to change or increase the pain relief you are receiving.

CARING FOR YOUR BABY

The hospital stay marks the beginning of the long process of learning to care for your baby and to meet his physical and emotional needs. Because you are recovering from surgery and are in need of care yourself, you will be given some assistance in looking after your new baby. In the first few days when getting out of bed, standing, walking and lifting are difficult, you will need help in dressing your baby, washing him and changing his nappy. Initially, you will not be able to lift him out of his cot unaided, so he will need to be passed to you to be fed. The important subject of breastfeeding after a caesarean is discussed in some detail in Chapter 6.

Many of us find that it takes us slightly longer than other mothers to become confident in handling and looking after our babies, particularly if we are first-time mothers. But as we recover and are able to do more for our infants, so we gain in confidence, and by the time we leave hospital we are invariably as competent as any other new mother.

The amount of help given to caesarean mothers appears to vary enormously. It is clear that some caesarean mothers are not receiving all the assistance they need in caring for their babies:

> When my baby was less than twenty-four hours old I was expected to care for him unaided. I was offered no help and had to try and get out of bed to feed and change him both day and night. After a further thirty-six hours I begged the night staff to take him into the nursery. They refused saying they weren't there to look after the babies!

Whilst all caesarean mothers need and deserve some help in the first few days, it is also vitally important that we participate in the day-to-day care of our babies as much as we are able, for it is out of such care that confidence and love develop:

> I can only praise the staff who gave me the right balance of support yet encouraged independence and mobility.

Many hospitals have a policy of taking caesarean babies into the nursery, for the first night at least, to help us to get a good night's sleep. Although this policy is well-intentioned, and much appreciated by some caesarean mothers, many of us find that we simply lie awake missing our babies and wondering if they are awake or crying. You have every right to keep your baby with you at night, and blanket policies that fail to take account of individual women's preferences are not helpful. This mother wrote:

> I kept my baby with me at all times. I needed her with me because I needed to reassure myself at a glance that it had indeed all been worthwhile.

A few hospitals now encourage new mothers to take their babies into bed with them — something that many caesarean mothers would appreciate:

My baby was left sleeping in bed with me and the staff rolled me over on my side to feed him during the night. They would come and tuck us both in so we didn't fall out.

It is, however, inadvisable to sleep with your baby if you have taken sleeping tablets, or recently had an injection of Omnopon or pethidine, or if you are still feeling groggy after a general anaesthetic.

The hospital staff are not the only ones who can help you to care for your baby. Your partner can also be invaluable in this respect. Most hospitals place very few restrictions on how long partners can stay, and it is a great help if your partner is able to be with you for most of the day. Whilst most caesarean mothers greatly appreciate their partner's visits, this is not always the case with other visitors. You may enjoy the company of visitors and showing off your new baby, but if you are too tired or do not feel like having them around it is important to say so. Good friends and close relatives should understand and are unlikely to be offended.

A significant minority of caesarean babies have to spend some time being looked after in the special care nursery. You will of course still be involved in the care of your baby — feeding him, caressing him and looking after him in other ways. This special situation is discussed more fully in Chapter 6.

ON AN EMOTIONAL ROLLERCOASTER

During our stay in hospital many of us feel as if we are riding on an emotional rollercoaster. We may feel euphoric at times, and only moments later feel helpless and despairing:

I was emotionally very labile. I sometimes cried with joy and wonder and sometimes with acute tiredness and feeling very sorry for myself.

I can remember telling one of my visitors that I would gladly have ten caesareans, and yet there were other days when I was crying for hours on end.

Many of us find it difficult to feel incapacitated, and feel frustrated at our physical limitations:

I felt so helpless and hopeless after the birth.

I remember feeling extremely envious of 'normal' mums, walking about with their babies, whilst I couldn't even pick myself up off the toilet!

Often what upsets us most is the fact that we are so limited in what we can do for our babies in the first few days:

I never even saw any of the first black [meconium stained] nappies as the nurses changed her in her cot which I couldn't see. It seems silly, but this upsets me.

In addition, many of us find it hard to ask for all the help we need, especially if the staff are very busy:

I remember I felt such a nuisance having to ask for help all the time.

On one occasion I lay for an hour watching my baby as he lay in his cot, wanting desperately to touch him, but was not quite able to reach. I didn't feel able to press my call button for such a supposedly minor reason as wanting to touch my baby.

Conflicting advice — about breastfeeding, babycare and what you are and are not able to do — can also be upsetting. On top of this, it is during our stay in hospital that we must confront the scar and begin to adjust to our new body image:

The bandage was removed on the second day and until about a week after I was scared of looking at the scar. When I eventually had the courage to look I was shocked at how large the scar seemed, but now fifteen months on it is very neat.

Perhaps the majority of caesarean mothers feel very tearful at some point during their hospital stay, particularly around four or five days after the birth. This weepiness is known as the maternity blues or the baby blues, and is experienced by up to 80 per cent of all new mothers. Although the maternity blues are often thought to be caused by fluctuating hormones after childbirth, there is, in fact, very little evidence to support this view, despite extensive biochemical investigation.[8] Some researchers feel that the baby blues bear more similarity to the 'end phenomenon' — the crying, anxiety and depression which often occurs after any period of intense stress.[9] This interpretation is further borne out by the fact that crying and depression are also very common after all forms of surgery, and are indeed even more common than the baby blues.[10] After a caesarean, we have both given birth and undergone major surgery, so it is not surprising that many of us feel very weepy at this time.

Although the maternity blues are common, it is important that our tears are not dismissed as 'just the blues':

> I felt very alone and frightened and cried at night — a nurse said, 'Oh, baby blues, I see, go back to sleep, you'll feel better' — how would I ever cope?

There is often meaning behind the tears. Any birth is a major life event and the arrival of a new baby alters a woman's life irrevocably in both positive and negative ways. There are many things about caesarean birth, as discussed in Chapter 3, that can be disturbing and distressing. There are aspects of the hospital stay that are upsetting. As well as all this, there is ample evidence that tearfulness is considerably aggravated by exhaustion and lack of sleep.[11] These feelings and experiences need to be acknowledged and accepted rather than brushed aside as merely the baby blues.

COMING HOME

The normal stay after a caesarean can vary by anything from five to ten days after the birth. When you are discharged will depend on the typical practice in your hospital, on how quickly you recover and on whether both you and your baby are well. Most good hospitals will also take your views into account: some women are very keen to go home as early as possible, others like to remain in hospital for the maximum stay. When you feel ready to come home will depend on the amount of support and rest you are getting in hospital, and on the amount of help you have lined up for when you come out. If you have your partner at home and your family close by to help then you may well find that an early discharge is best. If you will have to cope largely on your own a later discharge is probably more sensible.

You have the right to discharge yourself from hospital. In my research, one woman discharged herself after four days, another after just two days. You may be asked to sign a form stating that you discharged yourself against medical advice. You and your baby are nevertheless still entitled to the care of a community midwife who is obliged to visit you at home on a daily basis until at least ten days after the birth.[12]

After leaving hospital you will be looked after by the community midwife and by your GP and health visitor, care which the majority of caesarean mothers find adequate. However, the system does not always work well:

> I had a different community midwife every day, all of whom gave conflicting advice and seemed in a hurry, and I felt very unsupported.

In fact around one third of the women in my research felt that they did not receive enough support from the medical professionals caring for them once they left hospital.

When you are discharged from hospital you may be given specific instructions about activities to be avoided for certain lengths of time, but it is quite common for caesarean mothers to be given no guidelines whatsoever, or to receive the bland advice to 'take things easy'. Consequently, some women undertake too much too soon after a caesarean and end up taking longer to recover from the birth than they might otherwise have taken. Basically, it is important to be guided by your own body, and if in doubt ask your midwife or doctor. It can also be helpful to remind yourself (and those around you) that people undergoing operations similar to caesareans are advised to take as much as three months off work.

It is important to avoid heavy lifting during the first few weeks after a caesarean. This is easier said than done if you have a toddler as well as your new baby to care for. You should also try to avoid any housework that involves lifting, pushing or stretching for the first four to six weeks. This includes hoovering, ironing, carrying heavy shopping bags or laundry and changing beds. Your partner, family or friends may be able to help with these tasks. Caesarean mothers also sometimes receive the services of a home help for a short period after the birth. This can be arranged through your health visitor or GP, and, although provision is somewhat patchy, it is certainly worth asking about.

In addition to limiting the amount of housework you do, it is a good idea to try to set aside some time each day to have a rest.

You may be advised not to drive for the first two to six weeks after the birth. This is because the seat belt might irritate your scar and you may still be feeling weak and less able to respond to a sudden emergency properly. Some women can find this restriction very frustrating:

I was physically limited by the caesarean. I couldn't drive for six weeks, certainly couldn't lift a pram on and off buses and trains and even levering the pram up and down curbs pulled on my stomach. Carrying my daughter in a sling also hurt my stomach and so I certainly felt isolated at home. I felt very sorry for myself.

There is no recommended minimum time limit to keep to before resuming love-making. This depends entirely upon how you feel. Some women feel like making love a couple of weeks or so after a caesarean:

A lot of people talk about leaving sex for months, while we returned to normal (with care) within a fortnight — although it did hurt a little — but after a month it was just like before!

One nice thing, because it wasn't a vaginal birth, our sex-life was unaffected, no waiting for months and strain building up between you. One of my first conscious thoughts was 'at least I don't have to go through all that again!'.

Other women do not feel up to sex for a few months. This may be because they feel too tired or do not feel physically well enough:

My scar was very tender for a while and I was so tired for the first couple of months I didn't feel like sex.

We didn't resume love-making until three months after the op, I was experiencing pain up to seven months after delivery, and still even now [more than a year after the birth] have to adopt certain positions which are more comfortable.

Sex should not be painful after a caesarean, especially after the initial tenderness in the scar has worn off. If you find intercourse painful it is a good idea to mention this to your GP as you may have a lingering infection or some other problem that needs treating.

For some women it can take a long time to feel emotionally ready to resume love-making after a caesarean — this is discussed in Chapter 5. Sometimes it is the partner's emotional reaction to the caesarean that holds up a couple's sex-life, a situation which is discussed in Chapter 7.

Again there are no set guidelines about when it is safe to resume exercising after a caesarean, since this will depend on how much exercise you did before the birth, and on your rate of physical recovery. Like any other newly-delivered mother you will either be taught some postnatal exercises whilst in hospital or will be given a sheet of paper describing these exercises when you are discharged. Exercises to be done after a caesarean are very similar to ordinary postnatal exercises, but you should do them at your own pace, and do not push yourself too hard too soon. Pelvic floor exercises are also important after a caesarean since your pelvic floor will have been stretched during pregnancy. Swimming is an excellent form of post-caesarean exercise which can safely be resumed after your six-week check-up.

This six-week postnatal check-up is sometimes carried out by your GP, and sometimes by a doctor at the hospital where your baby was born. If you have not received a full explanation of the reasons for your caesarean by the time you are discharged from hospital, the six-week check-up is a good opportunity to discuss this. It is important that you find out not only why your caesarean was carried out, but also what is likely to happen in future births.

You may be sent to have a pelvic x-ray at this time, but policies vary. Some hospitals routinely x-ray all women who have had caesareans while they are still in hospital, some do this at the six-week check and others only x-ray when events in labour suggest disproportion. There are also some doctors who do not recommend pelvic x-rays after a caesarean since such x-rays are relatively poor at predicting whether a vaginal birth will be possible in future and are unlikely to alter decisions about subsequent deliveries. Some women are keen to have a pelvic x-ray, since in some cases it can help to provide some answers as to why a caesarean was necessary, and may give some indication of the chances of a caesarean being necessary in future births. If you feel this way and are not offered an x-ray, it is well worth asking for one. Equally, you are under no obligation to have an x-ray, if you do not wish to be x-rayed or do not feel that it would be helpful in your case.

PHYSICAL RECOVERY

Rates of physical recovery after a caesarean vary enormously from woman to woman, and it is very difficult to specify how long each stage of recovery will take, but I will attempt to give some guidelines. The initial pain in your scar usually wears off quickly after the first couple of weeks. After that you are likely to feel some discomfort in your scar, especially when bending, lifting or pushing, and at night when lying in one position often pulls on it, but this gradually diminishes and after a couple of months you will probably feel no discomfort there whatsoever. A minority of women nevertheless report feeling occasional twinges in their scar months or years after the caesarean. However, if you are experiencing more than the occasional twinge, or the pain in your scar appears to be getting worse rather than better, you would be well advised to see your doctor to check that all is well.

The appearance of your scar will also change with time. It will change in colour from red to pink, and will eventually turn a silver or white colour. Sometimes part of the scar remains a darker colour. Caesarean scars often seem smaller after a while since it is the edges of the scar that tend to fade the fastest. Your scar may be raised to form a small ridge or it may be flat. In most cases, lower segment scars are hidden below the pubic hair, but this is not always so. Sometimes all or part of the scar is above the hairline, and sometimes scars are lopsided. Most women, however, do find that the appearance of their scar improves dramatically as their pubic hair grows back.

Some women find that their scar is itchy, occasionally even months or years after the birth. It is also not uncommon for parts of the flesh on either side of the scar to feel numb; sometimes this numbness disappears after a few weeks or months, sometimes it remains.

There is more to physical recovery than the healing of the caesarean wound. After major surgery most people find that they tire more easily, that they lack energy and feel somewhat weak and below par for some time. Some caesarean mothers feel physically recovered in around one month, but others report that it took them as much as two years to fully recover physically from caesarean childbirth:

It is eight weeks after his birth and I feel completely recovered.

I think the worst part of a caesarean birth is the long recovery afterwards, especially as you have a new baby to cope with. I found myself becoming depressed and very frustrated, not being able to do the housework and go out as much as I wanted to.

Generally, though, full physical recovery can be expected to take up to six months.

In most cases physical recovery is straightforward, but it can sometimes be marred by complications. Some types of complication are apparent immediately after the birth; if you have lost a lot of blood during the caesarean, for example, you may need a blood transfusion. This is often a relatively simple procedure, but it can be quite distressing:

I spent sixteen hours on a drip being transfused blood and saline solution. All I wanted to do was sleep. I felt chained to the bed and everyone but me was looking after my baby.

Spinal headaches, which can occur after both spinal and epidural anaesthesia, are another form of complication. Such headaches occur when the dura of the spinal column is punctured and some cerebrospinal fluid leaks out:

When I first got out of bed I was struck by the most excruciating headaches. I had considered these to be possible side-effects, but pain like this can hardly be shrugged off or dealt with any other way than staying flat in bed. Every trip to the toilet became an event to be put off as long as possible. After five days of this I had a blood patch [a procedure in which some of the woman's own blood is injected into the spine to form a clot to seal the hole in the dura] and like a miracle the headaches were cured within half an hour. I cried tears of relief.

If your caesarean was carried out after a failed forceps delivery you will have an episiotomy as well as a caesarean wound. One caesarean mother who experienced this described feeling that she had had the worst of both worlds, as if she had had the baby twice.

Wound infections are perhaps the most common complication of caesarean childbirth. Signs that wound infection may be present include a raised temperature, the wound being red or weepy, hard lumps developing behind the scar, increasing pain in the scar region or the wound opening slightly. Wound infections can manifest themselves as early as the day after delivery, during the hospital stay or a number of weeks after the birth. They are usually caused by airborne bacteria that enter the wound during the surgery, although sometimes the infection occurs later as bacteria from the outside enter the wound. Often wound infections are cleared up quickly and effectively by a short course of antibiotics, but occasionally infections can recur or be resistant to antibiotics and linger for several weeks or even months. Having a wound infection can be a relatively trivial event or it can be very painful and highly traumatic, depending on the nature of the infection:

My wound was infected less than twenty-four hours after the birth and my stitches came apart leaving me with an open wound and in complete agony.

I left hospital exhausted, with a wound infection that took two months to heal, a shadow of my former self.

It is not possible, or desirable, to describe here all the different complications that occasionally occur after a caesarean. All caesarean mothers who experience complications should be given a full explanation of their complication by the medical professionals caring for them. If such explanations are not forthcoming, it is important that you ask for all the information you need, since understanding the nature, cause and treatment of a complication makes it a lot easier to cope with.

THE FIRST STEPS TO EMOTIONAL RECOVERY

The wound in our mind can take a lot longer to heal than the wound on our body. Emotional recovery is also sometimes more complex than physical recovery. It can be described as a four-stage process that begins with a state of physical and emotional shock. This is followed by a period of denial, when women feel there is nothing to be upset about. After this comes a painful stage of sadness and anger. The final step to emotional recovery is one of acceptance and coming to terms with the whole experience.

It is important to emphasise that, although the majority of caesarean mothers go through a process of emotional recovery similar to that described here, there is immense variation in both the length of time each stage lasts and the intensity of the emotions experienced. In addition, some women skip stages or experience two stages at the same time. It is the first two stages that tend to be experienced during the hospital stay and the first few weeks at home.

Many caesarean mothers will recognise the feeling of shock that often occurs during the first days or weeks after the birth, particularly after an emergency caesarean. Feelings at this time have been described as a kind of immobilisation, a sense of being overwhelmed or frozen up:[13]

> I spent the first six weeks or so shaking with shock inside.

> I felt really strange for the first couple of days, sort of like I was dreaming it all, it was unreal and I felt out of touch. I don't remember a lot of what happened either.

When this sense of shock and unreality passes, many of us refuse to acknowledge that having a caesarean was in any way a difficult experience for us. Although it is true that, for some women, caesarean childbirth is indeed not a difficult experience, for others, this denial is a coping mechanism, a way of disassociating ourselves from the experience:

> It didn't strike me until quite a long time afterwards that I am in some ways upset about the caesarean.

> I remember thinking, 'Wouldn't it be awful if all this happened to somebody else, like a single parent or a 16 year old?' It wasn't until some time later that I could begin to think, 'Isn't it awful that all this has happened to me?'

This 'denial' may well be a healthy response because after a very distressing experience we may need to shield ourselves from the intensity of the emotional pain, just as we would initially shield our eyes from the bright midday sun.[14]

5 The Wound in the Mind

'And who sutures the wound in my mind?'
From the poem 'Once a Cesarean — Now What?' by Jami Osborne[1]

Having experienced the sense of shock and then denial that often occur in the early period after caesarean childbirth, we then enter the third phase of emotional recovery — the stage of sadness and anger. We begin to confront the complex mixture of feelings that are the emotional scars of caesarean birth, the 'wound in the mind'.

If you are presently facing a caesarean delivery, you may find that reading this chapter leaves you feeling concerned about how you are likely to feel after the birth. Caesarean mothers, myself included, are generally very reluctant to talk to pregnant women about the difficult feelings that can arise after a caesarean. But to be forewarned is to be forearmed — if you do experience feelings of sadness and anger, you will be prepared and will perhaps be able to make more sense of these feelings. At least you will know that you are not alone in feeling like this.

It is also important to realise that the difficult emotions described here are not necessarily all part and parcel of caesarean birth. Giving birth by caesarean can be a very positive and fulfilling experience. In fact, there are a number of things that you can do to help to make the experience a more positive one (some suggestions are given in Chapter 10). By preparing yourself, becoming informed and knowing what options are available to you, you are minimising your chances of experiencing some of the painful feelings described below.

Also, try to bear in mind the fact that very few of us will experience all the sad and angry feelings described in this chapter, and that our difficult feelings are usually intermingled with feelings of love for our babies and joy at their arrival.

Furthermore, how long these difficult feelings last, and how deeply they are felt varies considerably. For some women, feelings of sadness and anger are fleeting and transitory.

You may be reading this after a caesarean and find that you have not felt any of the difficult emotions I describe. If this is so, then you are fortunate, but you are certainly not alone in feeling this way:

> Many people say you do feel cheated by having a section — I didn't and I felt that perhaps there was something wrong with me because I didn't feel like that.

Some women do begin to feel that they must be abnormal for feeling positive about having a caesarean, and wonder whether perhaps they should be feeling upset about it. But there are no 'shoulds' and 'oughts' about emotions — what you feel is an equally valid response to caesarean childbirth, and certainly not one that you should feel pressured into denying.

For some women caesarean birth is indeed primarily a positive experience, whereas for others it is a highly distressing experience which leaves them in deep emotional pain that may last for months or even years. It is important to ask why this is, and to establish what it is that makes having a caesarean a positive or a negative experience.

A number of researchers have found that emergency caesareans are more difficult to cope with than those planned in advance.[2] Similarly, it is apparent that women are more likely to experience difficult feelings or unhappiness after a caesarean under general rather than regional anaesthesia.[3] In addition, it is clear from my own research that the way we feel after a caesarean is also influenced to a large degree by the factors described in Chapter 3 — how necessary we perceive the caesarean to have been, the extent to which we felt informed and involved in childbearing decisions and the amount and quality of the support we received before, during and after the birth.[4]

When women have feelings of sadness and anger about caesarean birth, these emotions can appear at any time after the birth. Sometimes they surface after a few days or weeks, but sometimes it is not until months or even years later that a woman experiences the emotional pain, as this women found:

In my labour report for our antenatal teacher I said that I would gladly have another caesarean, as long as I didn't have to go through the twelve hours of labour first! This attitude stayed with me for the next eighteen months. It wasn't until I was at a talk about water birth that a sudden sadness and longing hit me. Afterwards I talked to the woman giving the talk and a flood of bottled-up feeling and tears poured out.

It is not unusual for the sadness and anger to appear after months of positive feelings about the birth:

In the days following the section the sense of relief that the worst was over was overwhelmingly enormous, I was in a state of euphoria because I had survived my worst nightmare. This feeling of euphoria lasted for three or four months, about the time it took for life to settle into the new version of 'normality'. One day, out of the blue, like a slap in the face, with absolutely no warning, the thought struck — 'I have a baby, but I have never given birth'. Words cannot describe how deeply sad I felt. The sense of loss, failure, why me, where did I go wrong? Over the months I've cried and cried and cried. I thought perhaps if I cried enough I would not be able to cry any more. But the tears just keep coming.

There are certain times when our distress is most likely to surface. One of these times is when a close relative gives birth vaginally. Another vulnerable time for some women is on the baby's first birthday, when memories of the caesarean can come flooding back. But perhaps the time when we are most vulnerable to these feelings is when we subsequently become pregnant, a situation which is discussed in Chapter 9.

It is important to analyse our emotional pain and to consider what the sadness and anger is about. There appear to be five main issues around which difficult feelings revolve. These are the sense of loss; issues concerning our identity and the way we feel about ourselves; a questioning of our mortality; feelings of violation; and a sense of betrayal.

A LOSS TO BE MOURNED

All new mothers need to grieve to some extent, because the birth of a baby also involves many losses — the loss of pregnancy, the loss of the exclusive couple relationship, the temporary or long-term loss of employment and the loss of the imagined baby, since the baby in one's arms is often quite different from the *dream* baby that pregnant women fantasize about. When we give birth by caesarean we suffer all these losses but we also experience other losses particular to caesarean childbirth. These may include the loss of the idealised birth we had hoped for; the loss of labour; the loss of the experience of giving birth; the loss of the first moments of the baby's life; and the temporary loss of strength and energy that follows a caesarean. Consequently, some degree of sadness and anger is appropriate and often inevitable after a caesarean. Losses need to be mourned:

There was I feeling like someone or something had died.

During pregnancy we all hold fantasies about the impending birth, imagining how it might be, and creating an image of the sort of birth experience we hope for. It is rare for this imagined birth to be a caesarean. The greater the disparity between the birth we fantasize about and the actual delivery, the more keenly we feel the loss of our hopes for the birth:

One thing which still hurts are period pains because they feel like those early contractions which had been so full of hope.

It can be difficult to understand why women whose caesareans are carried out before the onset of labour may need to grieve for the loss of the experience of labour, since labour usually brings with it a fair amount of pain. Many people imagine that a women would be pleased, not sad, to have avoided labour. It is certainly true that some caesarean mothers feel this way, but this is not always the case. For many women, labour is an essential part of childbirth. It is a physical and emotional challenge that marks one of life's most momentous events. Although the pain of labour is intense, it is, for many women, a positive pain, somewhat like the pain involved in running a marathon or climbing a mountain. Most of us can understand why people run marathons, and how it would not be quite the same for the runner to simply catch a bus to the finishing line. A similar idea is conveyed in the poem 'A Labor Saving Device' by Joan Joffe Hall.[5] Here she conjures up surreal images of people being knocked unconscious and carried to the movies, the circus or a basketball game, to save them the 'hassle' of getting there under their own steam. The poem ends with the poignant words 'That's just the way I had a baby'.

Many caesarean mothers also feel sad about not taking an active part in the birth of their children:

> I felt that the birth had been taken completely out of my hands. My body had not contributed in any way to my son's birth.

> So Alice was surgically removed from my body. And that is exactly how I felt. I have no feeling of having given birth.

American caesarean birth writers and campaigners, Nancy Cohen and Lois Estner, aptly wrote, 'If giving birth is like climbing a mountain, being sectioned is like being dropped off on the top of the mountain by helicopter. The view is the same, but for most women it *feels* different . . . What is different about the view is the *participation in the climb.* The sense of accomplishment and pride that accompanies a difficult task is missing. The "We did it, we really did it!" feeling.'[6]

For some women, the feeling of 'not giving birth' is one of the most difficult aspects of caesarean childbirth:

> Basically I feel as though I spent a long time baking a very special cake, then through no fault of anyone, someone else had to come along, take it out of the oven and ice it. Despite the fact that they did a beautiful job, I simply wanted to do it myself.

Others describe it as being like looking forward to Christmas all year long, only to wake up on Boxing Day to find that it is all over and someone else has opened your presents. Even those who have regional anaesthesia and so do participate in the birth can feel a sense of loss:

When my sister-in-law recently gave birth 'normally', albeit hardly pain-free, I actually felt jealous of her because she had experienced the visual as well as the physical aspects of her baby being born.

When a caesarean is carried out under general anaesthesia the physical process of conception/pregnancy/birth/feeding and caring for the new baby is interrupted at its most crucial point. This lost hour or so can make it difficult to assimilate and integrate the whole experience, leaving women with a deep feeling that something is missing:

> I suppose I feel there I was one minute pregnant, a tiny life inside me, totally dependent on me, seeing, feeling baby kick, the next minute I'm in a hospital ward with baby in a crib and a feeling of not knowing how he got there and being totally out of control of the situation.

Perhaps the most devastating loss suffered by women who have had caesareans under general anaesthetic is not 'being there' when their baby enters the world, and the loss of the first moments of their child's life:

> I feel very sad that I have to try and imagine the most remarkable moments of my life that my friends will have with them for the rest of their lives.

> It hurts to see photos of newborn babies — my son had been cleaned up when I first saw him — I had been a midwife and it seemed unfair that of all the newborn babies I had seen, I hadn't seen my own.

> I feel I have lost out on the most important time with one's newborn baby, something that I can never have again, something that I will regret for the rest of my life.

Many women feel very sad that they were not there to greet their babies and welcome them into the world. Others feel upset that other people knew about the baby before they themselves came round from the anaesthetic:

I feel the birth was stolen from me — that everybody knew I had a daughter and what she looked like before I did.

Occasionally, particularly when women have suffered debilitating complications or postnatal depression, this sense of loss can extend well into the postnatal period, with caesarean mothers feeling that they have lost not only the first moments of their baby's life, but also the first days, weeks or even months of life with their new baby:

With my son's birth there is just a blank from the time I was taken in for the operation, to about a day later, as I was given pethidine after the operation, and I didn't really come round until they stopped giving it to me [this type of reaction is relatively rare]. Now I feel as if someone has taken away some of the most important hours of my life. After all, no matter how many children I have, I can't have him again — and I regret it bitterly.

I felt sad that I wasn't able to enjoy my baby as I felt too ill for the first four to five weeks.

I feel very bitter that I totally missed out on my son's first six months of life. My husband looked after him and I can honestly say that it took me well over a year before I felt anything like my old self.

All these losses may leave us with a profound feeling of having missed out. This feeling is often accompanied by an envy of women who have easy births with little medical intervention:

When I listen to the accounts of other women's births, I feel sad, angry and resentful. They had done what I hadn't been able to do. Women speak of the satisfaction and euphoria they experienced after the birth, something I completely missed out on. I recently saw a woman giving birth on television while I was breastfeeding. I burst into tears, because the film brought back all the anticipation and expectations of pregnancy, which never had a chance to come true.

I still cry uncontrollably when I see a natural birth and am envious of my friends talking of their labours. How do I ever get rid of these feelings of guilt, inferiority and the deepest, deepest feeling of having missed out?

ALTERED IDENTITIES

Caesarean birth can also alter the way we feel about ourselves, our very identity. The caesarean knife may even 'cut through to the core of our being'.[7] It can damage our confidence and self-esteem, leaving us with feelings of inadequacy and failure. It may also alter how we feel about ourselves as women, our female identity. Having a caesarean can also affect the way we feel about our body.

Some women experience a profound sense of failure after giving birth by caesarean:

I felt I had failed part of my basic being.

I really felt I had let myself down as a mother in not being able to give birth vaginally.

I can still recall all the details of my feelings as though it was yesterday. I felt I'd failed.

Feelings of failure seem to be more common after long and difficult labours and when caesareans are carried out for reasons such as failure to progress. These feelings are often accompanied by self-blame, when women reproach themselves for having had a caesarean, or feel guilty about what they did or did not do during pregnancy or labour:

I felt cheated by having had a caesarean but quite appreciated that I couldn't have done it myself — after all they left me for hours and hours and I proved I was no good.

I sometimes think I didn't try hard enough.

He tried to induce me but I failed to dilate at all. I felt so useless. I'd been given such a good chance of a vaginal delivery and had mucked it up.

Sometimes women find themselves attempting to compensate for the feelings of failure they experienced after the caesarean:

When I was at home I had terrible feelings of inadequacy, that I hadn't been able to have a 'normal' delivery, and that I then had to be extra good at everything else to make up for this failure. I used to carry my son in his buggy up four floors to prove to everyone how fit I was.

Caesarean childbirth can also damage our feelings about ourselves as women, leaving us feeling somehow less feminine. For some women, reproductive capabilities are peripheral to their sense of identity as women, but for others they are central. Whilst most people can understand and sympathise with the way a vasectomy or impotency may affect a man's sense of male identity and his feelings of masculinity, many people find it difficult to understand why a woman might feel less womanly after a caesarean birth.[8] But giving birth is often an integral part of our sexual identity. It is, in some sense, what defines and unites us as women and differentiates us from men. Consequently, 'not giving birth' can have a deep and lasting effect:

I felt, and still do to some extent, that I failed as a woman. Giving birth is supposed to be the most natural thing for a woman to do — but I couldn't do it.

I felt a great sense of failure and less of a woman.

For God's sake, every woman who's half a woman can have children, so where did that leave me?

Caesarean birth can affect not only the way we perceive ourselves as women, but also sometimes how we see ourselves as mothers:

It all came to a head when my mother-in-law and my friend were arguing between them about how much milk my son should have, and I said, 'Don't mind me, I'm only his mother,' and my mother-in-law said, 'But you're not his mother. You never gave birth to him. You took the easy way out, you just lay there and did nothing.' I tried to explain that I had given birth to him, that I'd wanted to give birth naturally, but it was too dangerous, and why did it matter how he'd arrived anyway, and that I'd cared for him for eight months and loved him, but the words wouldn't come out. Deep down I agreed with them.

A woman's confidence in her body and feelings of wholeness and normality may also be sorely challenged by a caesarean birth, leaving her feeling abnormal, an oddity. These women wrote:

I thought I must be a real freak.

I blamed myself for being a physical failure as a mother, bodily deformed so that I couldn't produce my child like a real mother would.

Feelings such as these are more common after a caesarean carried out for disproportion. To tell a woman that she has an 'inadequate pelvis' or that there is no way that she could deliver a normal size baby can be very damaging psychologically. Such statements may also be medically incorrect, since there have been a number of cases where women who have been told that they have an inadequate or contracted pelvis have gone on to give birth vaginally to average or even large babies.[9] The question of pelvic size and future deliveries is discussed further in Chapter 9.

INTIMATIONS OF MORTALITY[10]

So far all the painful feelings I have described relate to birth, but a caesarean delivery is not just a birth, it is also an operation, and surgery brings with it another set of difficult emotions.

An operation, particularly a major operation, is an event that often causes individuals to confront their own mortality for the first time. Of course, we all know that one day we will die but for most of us this knowledge remains somewhat abstract and unreal. It is often not until we are in a situation that presents some perceived degree of risk that we come face to face with the fact that life is temporary. Some caesarean mothers become preoccupied with mortality statistics. Others find themselves wondering what would have happened if they had given birth a hundred years ago — would the baby have died? Would they have died? Watching operations on television is sometimes upsetting:

> Mentally I felt I put up a lot of barriers just before and during the operation. I didn't dare think about what was happening. Afterwards I found the sight of operating theatres on TV made me shudder for quite a long time.

Something else that is quite common after surgery, particularly after an emergency operation or one that results in complications, is the feeling that life itself is a risky and unpredictable business. Feelings of insecurity and vulnerability can be exacerbated by the fact that operations necessarily involve the violation of body boundaries. This can be particularly distressing when the psychological boundary between ourselves and others is weak, for physically-intrusive events like surgery can challenge this inner psychological boundary.[11]

In addition, being under general anaesthesia is sometimes likened to a mini-death, since the anaesthetised patient cannot see, hear or feel anything, and is unable to move or even breathe independently. This state of almost non-being can be very frightening for some women, and may provoke further reflections on death and mortality. Indeed, general anaesthesia has been referred to as the 'nearest brush with death that most of us experience in our lives'.[12]

Sometimes we are confronted by the realisation of our mortality directly, but sometimes our fears are apparent only in our dreams:

> A few months after the caesarean I had a dream in which I saw the body of a woman lying at the bottom of a lake. She was naked and heavily pregnant. She had been murdered and the stab wound ran across her lower abdomen.

VIOLATION

In the dream recounted above, associations are made between caesarean birth and, not only death, but also assault. This connection between surgery and assault is also made in Margaret Atwood's fictional account of a woman facing a mastectomy: 'She had a horror of someone, anyone, putting a knife into her and cutting some of her off, which is what it amounted to no matter what they called it. She disliked the idea of being buried one piece at a time instead of all at once, it was too much like those women they were always finding strewn about ravines or scattered here and there in green garbage bags.'[13]

In particularly difficult caesarean experiences, women write of feeling 'butchered' or even 'mutilated':

It was like being a piece of meat in a butcher's shop.

At times I felt outraged by the fact that someone had cut into my hitherto unscarred body and somehow violated me.

Sometimes, women describe their experiences as a form of torture:

I was given an excruciatingly painful internal examination, there seemed to be tubes and needles inserted all over my body, my pubic hair was being attacked by a razor blade — I felt totally bewildered, afraid and vulnerable. I felt as though I was being tortured, lying flat and vulnerable on a table and being attacked from every side.

Others who have had particularly bad caesarean experiences describe it as like being raped:

I felt almost raped, totally violated.

Childbirth educator Sheila Kitzinger has also drawn the analogy between difficult, disempowering birth experiences and rape.[14] She points out that women sometimes use the same words to describe how they felt during childbirth as those used by rape survivors, and may recount the same feelings of helplessness, depersonalisation and self-blame that are common after rape.

Caesarean mothers may also feel that their bodies have been damaged, and may take a long time to accept their new body image. Women's feelings about their caesarean scars vary considerably. Some women view their scar positively, others have no particular feelings about it, and some view it with intense dislike. Sometimes difficult feelings about the caesarean scar arise from the fact that not all scars correspond to the textbook description of a 'thin white line hidden beneath the pubic hair'. We are exhorted to see our scar as a 'smile', but to some women it can seem more like a gawping, hip-to-hip grimace:

> I lay there like an unfinished Bride of Frankenstein with fourteen metal clips holding my innards in place.

Sometimes women dislike their scar because they perceive it as a symbol or reminder of the whole caesarean experience. We may find it difficult to look at the scar, to touch it or to be touched there.

It is not surprising that negative feelings about the scar and a poor self-image often have a bad effect on the sex-lives of caesarean mothers. These women said:

> My scar is very depressing. I felt that my husband could not possibly find me attractive anymore (although I know he does). I have absolutely no self-confidence now, and getting into the bath used to make me feel utterly sick — I hated to be alone with my naked body. At 23 I felt like an old, ugly, repulsive hag.

> Although my scar has healed well I do not feel attractive and despite my husband's assurances that it makes no difference to the way he feels about me, I am conscious of my scar when I am naked and when we make love.

A SENSE OF BETRAYAL

For some women the difficult emotions that surface in this third stage of the caesarean experience centre on feelings of betrayal, and of having been let down. Anger is typically and in many instances justifiably focused on the hospital and medical profession:

> I frequently had nightmares and often awoke in the night wanting to smash windows at the hospital.

It is not uncommon for these feelings to occur several months after the birth. Indeed, as Nancy Stewart has pointed out, women's satisfaction with the medical treatment they received during childbirth tends to decrease over time, so that months later they may be very critical of interventions which they were grateful for immediately after the birth.[15]

For some women the sense of betrayal stems from feeling that their caesareans were unnecessary or avoidable:

> I kept wondering whether the operation could have been avoided and what would have happened if I hadn't consented to it. If I had chosen a consultant with a low caesarean birth rate, would the outcome have been different?

> What I found really upsetting about my caesarean was that I was not given a *chance* to go into labour, and that (as was afterwards admitted) it may not have been necessary after all.

> I feel cheated. I know I could have delivered her myself as she wasn't a big baby.

For some mothers, the anger is more about their lack of involvement and the way decisions were made over their heads. Such treatment can be very hurtful, for as psychoanalyst Joan Raphael-Leff points out, 'Even in an emergency, respect for the patient comes across, as does high-handed disregard. In obstetrics, as in any other professional contact, trust is the essence of client confidence in the practitioner. Unfortunately in some hospitals trust has been eroded by medical mystification, routine practices and authoritarian non-explanatory control.'[16]

For other women, it is the lack of support that leaves them feeling angry and upset:

In spite of the whole nightmare I did try to be co-operative with the hospital staff, but I feel they betrayed our trust and made an awful situation absolutely unbearable by treating us in such an unfeeling manner.

I felt really let down by my stay in hospital, as it was a time when I really needed a lot of support, but got very little. It made me feel as if I didn't matter at all.

POST-TRAUMATIC STRESS

Having a caesarean can be a very traumatic event, and some caesarean mothers find that they experience post-traumatic stress. Post-traumatic stress disorder is a well documented psychological reaction to disasters and other highly distressing events. It is now recognised that post-traumatic stress can occur after medical procedures as well as external events.[17] It manifests itself in several ways — sometimes people re-experience the event with vivid flashbacks, they may have difficulty in getting to sleep or may have nightmares, they may be irritable or startle easily and they may feel numb or withdrawn. One woman said:

When I went to bed I relived the whole experience every night for months until the details faded.

Another woman wrote four months after her caesarean:

This whole experience seems to haunt me. When I lie in bed, driving the car, shopping, anything, I get flashes back to the labour ward, the recovery ward. Although they are not frightening they will not leave me. I feel almost as if I cannot cope with it anymore.

But perhaps more common than post-traumatic stress, is postnatal depression.

POSTNATAL DEPRESSION

Postnatal depression can set in when the sad and angry feelings described in this chapter remain unexpressed and are turned inwards onto the self, or when these feelings are simply overwhelming. Postnatal depression may be defined as any form of prolonged depression that occurs in the first year following childbirth. Although estimates vary, it is thought to affect around 10 per cent of all mothers.[18] It is distinct from the 'baby blues', the tearfulness that occurs four or five days after the birth, which was discussed in Chapter 4. One woman who experienced depression following the caesarean birth of her daughter described the symptoms of postnatal depression as follows:

> . . . total exhaustion, so much so that you wake up in the morning as tired as when you went to bed; no energy, even filling a kettle with water wears you out; despair, nothing seems to be right, you look back to the golden days before you had the baby; no confidence in yourself as a mother or a person, everyone else around seems to be coping better than you; and panic attacks, before doing things like stepping out of the front door, shopping, visiting somebody — all situations you did not give a second thought to before you had the baby.

The exact relationship between caesarean birth and postnatal depression is unclear. A number of studies have failed to find a link between the two.[19] But this is perhaps not surprising, since postnatal depression is a complex phenomenon that may arise from the demands and isolation of motherhood, from disadvantaged social and financial circumstances, from the resurfacing of difficult feelings stemming from the woman's own childhood or from hormonal disturbances, as well as from difficult birth experiences. In addition, the circumstances of a caesarean birth can vary enormously — for some women the caesarean experience is truly depressing but for other caesarean mothers this is not the case at all. It is also important to realise that not all vaginal births are positive experiences. Therefore, a woman who has had a caesarean under optimal conditions will, in all probability, be less likely to experience postnatal depression than a vaginally delivered woman who felt alienated from and unsupported in her birth experience. To find the connection between difficult birth experiences and postnatal depression, it is not enough to simply count the number or type of interventions and to see if this is related to later depression — it is the quality of the experience that counts.

This is not to say that caesarean birth is not a contributory factor in postnatal depression — in some instances it clearly is. A number of studies have indeed found an increased incidence of postnatal depression following caesarean birth.[20] It is also true that many women who become depressed after birth perceive their caesarean to be an important factor in the genesis of their depression. I found that it was those women who had emergency caesareans, for whom it was their first caesarean, and who felt unsupported during the birth and the hospital stay, who were most likely to report having suffered from postnatal depression.[21]

Sometimes the depression begins within days of the birth:

Physically it was a 'textbook' caesarean. However, it was an emotional disaster. I was postnatally depressed and spent the first few weeks of my daughter's life shut up in my bedroom crying: I couldn't face anyone, and the baby was brought to me to be fed and then (if I could help it) whisked off again. Once my partner went back to work things got worse: I dreaded the baby's crying and would scream at her 'I hate you! I wish I had never had you!' when she cried for a feed. All I wanted to do was go back to work and get back to 'normal' — I felt the whole thing had been an awful mistake.

In other cases, postnatal depression surfaces gradually and incipiently, and emerges months after the birth. Sometimes the depression is hidden, which can make the sufferer feel even more isolated in her experience:

My recovery took a long time. Outwardly I appeared normal. I returned to work. I organised school visits by NCT members. I was amazed that I could talk sensibly in reply to questions about caesareans, while lying awake at night crying over the reality of my caesarean. There were two occasions when I felt like killing myself, and most of the time I wished I had not woken up after the operation, as it would have been much less trouble for everyone, especially me. None of my friends really guessed that I was screaming inside while smiling outside.

Now that I am well, I feel almost embarrassed that I was ever like this, but I suspect that others have felt similarly.

It is important to point out here that not all those who experience feelings of sadness and anger following a caesarean birth are suffering from postnatal depression. Some degree of grief and mourning are almost inevitable, and may even be a healthy reaction to the trauma of caesarean birth. For as Claudia Panuthos writes, 'The hurts that are present are not a sign of insanity, but rather a testimony to aware, awake mental health.'[22]

There is also a danger that in labelling the legitimate feelings of sadness and anger that often follow caesarean birth as postnatal depression, a woman's experience may be trivialised, dismissed and pathologised away. Our sadness and anger is meaningful and important. Experiencing and expressing these difficult emotions is all part of the process of coming to terms with a distressing caesarean experience. Ultimately we may emerge from our emotional pain having learnt and grown from the whole experience.

6 Mother and Child

BONDS OF LOVE

When you meet your newborn you may fall in love with her instantaneously. Many caesarean mothers report feeling this rush of love as they hold the new baby for the first time:

> As for bonding with my baby, I couldn't love her any more than I already do — and I love her with a powerful force nothing could compare with — and this feeling began from the second I held her.

There is a myth that bonding — the technical term for falling in love with our babies — is inevitably difficult after a caesarean, but this is certainly not always so. We have undergone surgery for the sake of our infants and this is, in itself, a profound act of love. Moreover, the relationship between mother and child is sometimes stronger because of the caesarean:

> Bonding, if anything, has been more ferocious on my part. I am anxious to show my son that I am his mum, even though I wasn't there at the birth (if you see what I mean).

However, this is not the case for all caesarean mothers and their babies. We do not yet know what effect, if any, caesarean birth has on the bonding process. It is certainly true that, in some species of animal, females delivered by caesarean sometimes show less maternal behaviour towards their offspring, although such behaviour is usually delayed rather than absent.[1] But we are very different from rats and sheep whose behaviour is largely instinctual, and to extrapolate from animal to human behaviour would be most unwise. Researchers who have observed caesarean-delivered and vaginally-delivered mothers and their infants report mixed findings. Some researchers have indeed found that caesarean delivery can have a deleterious effect on the mother-infant relationship.[2] In other studies, however, caesarean mothers were found to be no different from other mothers in the way they interact with their infants,[3] and in the way they feel about the baby.[4] In one study, caesarean mothers even received higher ratings on the quality of mother-child interactions than the vaginally-delivered mothers.[5] It seems that when caesarean birth does affect the relationship between mother and baby, the effects tend to be confined to the early period after the birth, and are probably largely due to pain and fatigue.[6]

Around one fifth of the caesarean mothers in my research reported experiencing some difficulty in forming a relationship with their baby.[7] When this happened it was usually the case that feelings of love were somewhat late in arriving, but when they did arrive these feelings were as deep as the feelings any other mother has for her child:

> I certainly didn't feel a great love for my baby straight away. I was pleased I'd got him and that he was OK, but didn't have the feeling of elation that some people talk about. It took a couple of weeks before I really felt as though I loved him.

It is also important to realise that by no means all vaginally-delivered mothers experience great feelings of love for their infants the moment they emerge from the womb. In one study, 40 per cent of first-time mothers recalled that their predominant emotion when holding their babies for the first time was one of indifference.[8] Other researchers found that a third of the mothers they studied reported that it was at least a week before they felt love for their babies.[9]

Occasionally, however, caesarean birth does give rise to difficulties in the relationship between mother and baby that may last for several months, just as it did in this case:

> I could not identify with the baby. For the first three months I was very impatient with her and fed her without looking at her. Luckily, I realised I was rejecting her and made an effort

to look at her and to talk to her. The breastfeeding helped a lot. Now at nine months I am beginning to love her a bit.

I found that women were more likely to have problems in forming a relationship with their babies when the caesarean was carried out under general anaesthetic; when it was an emergency caesarean; when the woman felt unsupported during the birth and while in hospital; and when she felt uninvolved in and uninformed about decisions taken during labour and delivery.[10] Such problems also seem to be confined to first caesareans, since it was very rare for women to report experiencing any difficulty relating to their babies after a second or subsequent caesarean.[11]

There is some evidence that it is the length of time that the mother and baby are separated after the birth, rather than the mode of delivery itself, that is the most important factor that influences the early mother–child relationship.[12] Researchers Marshall Klaus and John Kennel suggest that the first few hours after birth are a very special time for developing the bond between parents and baby — a time which they call the maternal sensitive period.[13] When a mother and baby are separated after the birth, as is the case with caesareans under general anaesthesia and when babies are taken into special care, then this period for early bonding is missed. The significance of this is unclear, since it is not yet known exactly how long this sensitive period lasts, and since it is apparent that very strong bonds of love can develop after long separations. Indeed, Klaus and Kennel strongly refute the notion that all is lost when long separations occur.[14] But what is so important about Klaus and Kennel's work is that they have highlighted that crucial time when parents meet their newborn. It is a time for what Sheila Kitzinger calls the emotional work of holding, exploring, touching and stroking the new baby, and of 'breathing in' his reality.[15]

This special time need not be foregone after a caesarean. All new parents should be given some time together, in privacy, with their new baby, to welcome him into the world and to begin their relationship as a family. Women who have had caesareans under general anaesthesia usually wake to find that their babies are fully dressed and cleaned up which makes the process of stroking and exploring the baby more difficult, but it does not have to be like this. In the American hospital where Klaus and Kennel work, babies born by caesarean are not dressed immediately after the birth. These babies are kept warm under a heat panel (if a heat panel is unavailable Klaus and Kennel suggest that, once dried, the baby could equally well be placed on his mother's chest with a warmed blanket placed over both of them) and the parents meet their baby in its unclothed 'newborn' state.[16] If you do miss out on this time after the birth you can have this special time during the hospital stay or when you return home:

> The sister came and said she was going to take my drip off. I said, 'Great, now if you don't mind I'm going to strip off and hold my baby close.' She was very good and understanding and left me in my room and drew the blind. Finally, after two and a half days, I was able to pick up my baby and hold him on my own.

BABIES IN SPECIAL CARE

A number of babies born by caesarean will need some form of special care. If your baby is very small she will need to be placed in an incubator to keep her warm. If she develops jaundice she may need to receive phototherapy. In some hospitals, incubators and phototherapy cots can be placed next to the mother's bed on the postnatal ward so that you and your baby do not need to be separated. If your baby has breathing difficulties at birth, if her lungs are not sufficiently mature to function without assistance, or if she is too weak to suck and feed, it will be necessary for her to receive special or intensive care in the special care baby unit. In my research, nearly a quarter of the babies received special care, sometimes for as little as one hour, sometimes for several weeks.[17] Babies born by caesarean are a little more likely to require special care since caesareans are often carried out because a baby is in difficulty — the baby may be distressed or premature — and because caesarean babies have a slightly increased risk of having breathing problems at birth (as discussed in Chapter 2). Thankfully babies are no longer routinely taken into special care after a caesarean delivery, although this does still happen in a small number of hospitals. This practice is deplorable and cannot be justified.

In most special care nurseries there is now a great sensitivity to the needs of new parents. You will be encouraged to visit as often and for as long as you like, to talk to, stroke and cuddle your baby, and to feed him. Babies who are too small, weak or poorly to breastfeed or to take a bottle are fed through a small tube which is passed through a nostril and down into the baby's stomach. This tube remains in place between feeds. If you wish to breastfeed, you will be encouraged to express your milk using a breast pump so that your baby can receive breastmilk via the tube, and to keep up your supply of milk so that you can breastfeed in the usual way once he is well enough.

Many of the women in my research could not praise the staff in the special care nursery highly enough, but a few felt very isolated from their babies, particularly in the first few days when caesarean mothers are not very mobile. It is particularly important for caesarean mothers not only to be able to be with their special care babies as much as possible but also to receive clear explanations of the reasons why special care is necessary and of the treatment that is given:

> I hated being separated from my baby after the birth, especially as no one told me why he was in special care.

Information, involvement and support can minimise the distress of parents whose babies need special care.

The feelings of loss that caesarean mothers sometimes experience about not seeing their babies in their newborn state are exacerbated for mothers of special care babies:

> I wish I could have seen him come into this world, all wet and slippery and naked. Instead, the first time I saw my baby, he was in an incubator, fully clothed, including bonnet and mittens, with tubes and bleeping machinery all around.

Sometimes when a baby needs to go into special care other relatives may be allowed to see the new baby before the mother herself does. This mother found it very hard:

The only real negative thing about my caesarean was that so many people saw my baby before I did. The first thing my mother said was 'I saw him before you did' and even now the thought upsets me. I didn't feel like his mum for a long time.

This can be very distressing and it would be helpful if hospitals adopted a policy of allowing no one, apart from the baby's father, to see or hold the baby before the mother herself is able to.

Because some degree of separation is inevitable when a baby needs special care, women sometimes find that it takes somewhat longer to feel love for their baby. But this is not always the case:

Finally, after two days I had actually seen, touched, held my baby. I loved him straight away.

In fact in my research those women whose babies needed special care were no more likely to report having difficulties in their relationship with their baby than other mothers,[18] which is perhaps a testament to the generally high standard of emotional care given by staff in special care nurseries.

Giving birth by caesarean and having a baby who needs special care are both difficult and challenging experiences. When a baby is born several weeks early, this adds a further complication to the emotional aftermath of caesarean birth:

I think in some ways the whole birth was full of shock, it being seven weeks early, that the caesarean was just another part of the whole nightmare for me — an almost predictable consequence when just about everything seemed to go wrong.

In a premature birth, as psychoanalyst Joan Raphael-Leff points out, 'nothing happens according to expectation and nothing is ready. The couple is caught unawares and usually the woman finds that the pregnancy has ended and labour begun before she has completed the emotional process of gradual separation.'[19]

This sense of shock may be compounded by the appearance of your premature baby, who will often look very different from the fantasy baby you imagined whilst pregnant:

The midwife wheeled him over so as I could see him. He was lying like a frog with spindly arms and legs covered in blond hair and looking a little unfinished.

Another particularly difficult aspect of having a premature baby is that you may return home before your baby is well enough to leave hospital, and this can be very hard:

My second baby was born eight weeks premature and had to go into special care. Coming home without her was the worst of all. I felt as if I had gone through the wars and lost everything.

In addition, when a baby is born very early there is an all pervading fear for the baby's life, and because of this parents are sometimes unsure about how involved they should allow themselves to become.

Many of the difficult feelings that can result from a caesarean birth that were described in Chapter 5 are also present when a baby is born prematurely — feelings of shock, loss, separation, guilt and failure. Bertrand Cramer, who has carried out a study of mothers of premature babies, writes, 'The pregnancy was not complete, the baby was not complete, and so many of these women concluded, irrationally, that they too were incomplete.'[20] If you have had a caesarean and your baby was born prematurely it is important that you, and others, recognise the enormity of what has happened to you, and that you give yourself the time and space to come to terms with the whole experience.

WHEN A BABY DIES

This chapter on caesarean birth and the mother–child relationship would not be complete without remembering that for some caesarean mothers there is no child. It is a sad fact that around one caesarean baby in 100 will die at or shortly after birth:[21]

As well as suffering grief, I felt a sense of guilt, failure and inadequacy and anger. Anger that we should have to lose our child with no control over her or our lives. Life is never certain and I try and treasure the moments we have.

To lose a baby is tragic. It has been described as an 'obscene contradiction'[22] and is the antithesis of all our expectations, for as Claudia Panuthos and Catherine Romeo write, 'The anticipation of life, of health, of birth is a stark contrast to the stillborn child or the infant who dies.'[23] The feelings of sorrow, guilt and anger, and profound grief, that parents experience when their baby dies can be overwhelming.

The long and painful process of coming to terms with such a loss is not helped by the fact that ours is a death-denying culture in which many people shy away from talking about death, creating almost a 'conspiracy of silence'.[24] If your baby has died you will need a lot of support, and may find it helpful to contact the Stillbirth and Neonatal Death Society (SANDS) whose address appears on page 238.

When a baby dies the sense of loss that many women feel after a caesarean is overshadowed by the much greater loss — the loss of the baby:

> I feel very sad that I went through a caesarean and then have no baby at the end of it. People say how they feel after a caesarean, but not many say they did not have any baby to help them get over it.

The effects of the caesarean may be forgotten and unacknowledged, but as Claudia Panuthos and Catherine Romeo point out, the caesarean is often very much a part of the total picture of birth-related loss, and complete emotional healing requires that the whole experience be mourned.[25]

BREASTFEEDING AFTER A CAESAREAN

Breastfeeding is an important part of the mother-child relationship. A study carried out in 1975 found that a mere 2 per cent of caesarean mothers breastfed their babies,[26] largely due to a lack of support and encouragement coupled with the expectation that women did not and could not breastfeed after a caesarean. The situation has improved dramatically since then. Many studies now report little difference in the numbers of caesarean-delivered and vaginally-delivered women who breastfeed,[27] and 80 per cent of women in my research breastfed their babies.

Breastfeeding can be of particular importance after a caesarean. It can help to promote feelings of love and attachment between mother and baby. Many women also find that breastfeeding is less tiring than bottlefeeding because it involves less work — there is no equipment to sterilise, no feeds to make up and no trips to the kitchen in the middle of the night to warm bottles. Breastfeeding is also very important during the early days when you need a lot of help in caring for your baby and can feel somewhat redundant — it is something that no one but you can do for her:

> I was extremely lucky in that I had no problems at all in breastfeeding. This was wonderful as it was something only I could do for my baby.

Breastfeeding can also help to restore feelings of confidence in your body and in your mothering abilities — confidence that may have been sorely challenged by the caesarean birth. When breastfeeding goes well it can also help to assuage the feelings of failure, and the damaged female identity that women sometimes experience after a caesarean. A number of caesarean mothers who breastfed their babies wrote 'at least I got something right'. But when breastfeeding does not succeed, for whatever reason, this can be a further devastating blow to a woman who feels that she has 'failed' by giving birth by caesarean:

> Because she had already been given a bottle and because it transpired I had flat nipples, I couldn't breastfeed. The feeling of failure was almost overwhelming. The thought that echoed around and around my head was I couldn't give birth to her properly and I can't even feed her — I am totally useless.

There is enormous variation in the timing of the first breastfeed after a caesarean. Many women who have caesareans with regional anaesthesia suckle their babies whilst still on the operating table. The baby is simply placed on your chest for his first nuzzle at your breast — something that most women find very satisfying. If you have a general anaesthetic it is still possible, with the assistance of a midwife, for your baby to suckle soon after his birth while you are still unconscious. Alternatively, you may wish to feed him soon after you awaken. But do not worry if you miss out on this early feed, for although many women enjoy it and feel that it helps to lay the foundations of successful breastfeeding, there is actually no evidence to suggest that if a mother does not feed her baby immediately after birth, then subsequent breastfeeding will suffer.[28]

In the early days after a caesarean you will need some help with breastfeeding. You will need someone to pass the baby to you, to arrange your pillows and help you to find a comfortable position. There are a number of different positions for breastfeeding after a caesarean, but the three positions most commonly used are shown in fig. 1.

In the lying-down position (fig.1a), you lie on your side with your lower arm outstretched above your baby's head or with your hand propping up your head, as illustrated. Lie your baby on a pillow, with her chest facing yours. To give the second breast, either place your baby on your chest and roll over onto your other side — you will need some help to do this at first. Or, rearrange the pillows (again you may need assistance) so that you can roll further over on the same side to reach your baby and offer her the second breast.

Another useful position for breastfeeding after a caesarean is the 'American football' hold, also known as the twins position (fig. 1b). You lie propped up with several pillows to support your back, while your baby lies on a pillow beside you with his body tucked underneath your arm. This position is particularly useful for feeding twins or small babies, or if you have a classical (vertical) scar.

You can also breastfeed sitting in a chair with your baby placed on one or two pillows on your lap (fig. 1c). This position is often more comfortable if you place a pillow behind you to support your back. If the chair is low it is helpful to sit on a pillow, if it is high you may find it more comfortable if you have a low stool for your feet to raise your lap.

Breastfeeding After a Caesarean

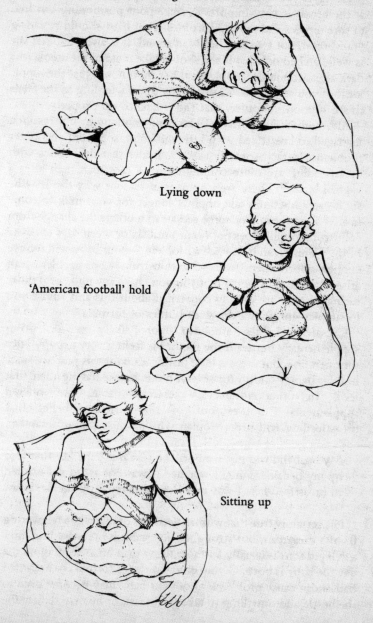

Lying down

'American football' hold

Sitting up

However you decide to breastfeed, the positioning of the baby at the breast is very important, since poor positioning can lead to sore nipples and other difficulties. Your baby should be facing your breast, not twisting her head round. It is also vital that she is well 'latched on', that is she should take most of the areola (the dark skin around the nipple) into her mouth, not just the nipple itself. If you see the top of your baby's ears wiggling as she feeds this is a good indication that she is latched on properly.

Although the majority of caesarean mothers in my research managed to breastfeed with little difficulty, some did encounter problems. In fact, some research indicates that difficulties with breastfeeding are more common after a caesarean than after a vaginal birth.[29] There are a number of reasons why this may be so. It can sometimes take slightly longer for your milk to come in after a caesarean. For some caesarean mothers the change from colostrum to milk does not occur until six or seven days after the birth.[30] This is rarely in itself a problem — your baby will receive enough nourishment from your colostrum — but problems can arise if you start to worry that you don't have any milk, or if those caring for you are unduly concerned about this and advise you to supplement your baby with bottles of formula.

Caesarean babies are also more likely to be given supplementary bottles if the mother is feeling very groggy after the operation, but there is little justification for this practice since healthy babies can go for several hours before having their first feed. In other instances, caesarean babies are offered supplementary bottles out of the mistaken belief that breastfeeding will tire a woman who has just had a caesarean:

> My husband was given a bottle to give our baby her first feed by my bedside, while I watched. I was not asked if I wanted to breastfeed her; I was told I couldn't try until the next day.

It is certainly true that women need lots of rest when recovering from a caesarean, but struggling to establish breastfeeding after a delayed start is usually far more tiring than breastfeeding on the day the baby is born. Giving extra bottles of formula to breastfed babies can cause problems since your baby may become used to the bottle and unwilling to take the breast, or he may reduce the amount of breastmilk he is taking which will diminish your supply. In fact, women whose babies receive supplementary bottles of formula are up to five times more likely to give up breastfeeding in the first week, and twice as likely to abandon it during the second week, than women whose babies are not supplemented and are encouraged to feel that their own colostrum and milk are adequate.[31]

There are other ways in which having a caesarean can give rise to breastfeeding difficulties. There are, for example, the after-effects of the operation itself:

> My grogginess interfered with the bonding process and made breastfeeding a struggle to establish, though we did get it going at last, and continued until quite recently [around eighteen months later] — perhaps by way of compensation.

Some women also find that having a caesarean takes away their confidence in their body and this may affect breastfeeding:

> One other worry, completely unfounded, was that I would have no milk, or be unable to feed; my body had already failed me once, so I no longer trusted it. In fact, feeding was so easy and blissful it seemed as if I'd spent all my life waiting to do it.

The ease with which you breastfeed after a caesarean may well depend on the amount of help and support you receive while in hospital. The right sort of help and advice can make all the difference:

> The nurses were fantastic helping me to breastfeed, something which I was quite determined to do, and they would come at any time to help.

But nearly one third of the caesarean mothers in my research felt that they did not receive enough help and support with breastfeeding;[32] inadequate help with breastfeeding appears to be a major dissatisfaction of all new mothers in hospital:[33]

> No one would ever stay with me for any length of time — they

would latch him on, go away and then I'd be left with him crying and me crying until someone eventually came back some time later. He'd always become 'unlatched' as soon as they went out of the door. I gave up after a week of trying.

If you do experience difficulties with breastfeeding, you may find it helpful to contact one of the breastfeeding support organisations listed on pages 237-8.

If you are bottlefeeding your baby after a caesarean there are a number of suggestions that you might find helpful. If you are finding it difficult to find a comfortable position to feed your baby, try one of the positions illustrated on page 121. It is important that it is you, rather than hospital staff or well-meaning relatives, who gives your baby her bottle most of the time, as feeding a baby is a special time which you will not want to miss out on. However, one benefit of bottlefeeding is that it is something that you can share with others such as your partner. Many caesarean mothers who bottlefeed particularly appreciate it if their partner takes over some of the night-time feeds, enabling them to get a good night's sleep. Finally, you might find it helpful to reorganise your home so that all that you need to make up bottles is close at hand, particularly at night, as this will minimise the amount of stair-climbing you need to do.

MATERNAL PERCEPTIONS

Here I would like to consider whether the way in which our children were born influences the way we perceive them. Do we see our children differently because they were born by caesarean? For some caesarean mothers this certainly seems to be the case.

For many, a caesarean baby is seen as a special baby. In ancient myths and legends, caesarean birth is believed to confer supernatural powers and to elevate those born in this way above ordinary mortals,[34] powers also attributed to Shakespeare's character Macduff in *Macbeth* who was 'from his mother's womb untimely ripp'd'. This idea receives some support from the work of psychologists Tiffany Field and Susan Widmayer, who found that mothers who have given birth by emergency caesarean tended to perceive their infants more positively and attributed them with more optimal characteristics than vaginally-delivered mothers.[35] They speculated that this may be because the emergency delivery is seen as a special or crisis event and consequently the emergency-delivered baby is viewed as special. Similarly, other researchers found that parents of caesarean-born children perceived their children to be more academically able than did the parents of vaginally-born children, despite the fact that the children did not differ in their actual ability.[36] In addition, the caesarean-born children themselves had higher expectations of their own academic performance.

Another common perception is that we have let our caesarean children down by not giving birth vaginally, and that consequently we feel sorry for them and feel the need to make reparations for the circumstances of their birth:

> I feel a complete and utter failure, and I feel sorry for James for having such a useless mum as me.

These feelings are more common after caesareans under general anaesthetic where invariably neither parent is 'there' to greet the newborn as she enters the world:

> In the hospital I remember just looking at her sleeping and shedding a few tears saying, 'Oh I'm so sorry I wasn't there with you, you were all on your own.' Then for months afterwards, every now and again, I used to cry, sometimes on my own, sometimes with my husband, because I missed being with her, she had been on her own and I hadn't been there to meet her.

> Instead of in my arms or at my breast in her early minutes of life, she was in a sterile cot. I feel I let her down and I am still trying to make it up to her. I hope some day I can.

Other women feel particularly sad about the effects that they perceive postnatal depression to have had on their children:

> What I am sorry about is the effect having the caesarean had on my daughter. Before I had my son [born vaginally] I used

to think that my unhappiness and postnatal depression hadn't had too bad a long-term effect. Now I can see how different motherhood (and babyhood) can be. It's a shame because we can never re-live that spoilt first year.

As my depression got worse I coped by looking after my son mechanically. It is only now that I realise how he must have missed out, and I try to make it up to him now. He means the world to me and I deeply regret that the circumstances of his birth had such an effect on his first year of life.

A number of caesarean mothers also described the disconcerting feeling that the baby was not really their own. When we have a caesarean under general anaesthetic we are unable to witness or experience the birth, and there may be a seed of doubt that the baby we meet when we regain consciousness is actually the baby that was inside us:

I am shocked when people say he looks like me, because in my subconscious there seems to be this belief that he is not mine. I love him dearly, absolutely, and yet there is still this amazement when anyone says he looks like me.

A regular nightmare was that she had been stolen and I couldn't prove she was mine. It is almost as if my baby died and someone said, 'Never mind, dear, have this one, it's better than the one you would have had anyway.' And yet I have no intellectual doubt that she is mine.

During one of the nights interrupted by trips to the nursery to feed the twins I dreamt I was breastfeeding puppies which didn't belong to me but to somebody who had appointed me as wet nurse. For weeks I couldn't quite imagine that these were the babies I had carried inside me for all those months. Maybe they were just given to me at birth? It only happened slowly and very gradually as they were growing and putting on weight as a result of my feeding and care, that I began to regard them as my own creations, my own babies.

This leaves some caesarean mothers feeling quite separate and detached from their babies:

> I have always seen her as a lovable, beautiful individual, not much to do with me. Her arrival had nothing to do with any conscious thought or action on my part. She wasn't born, she was cut out. I didn't give birth to her, I just happened to be there. She doesn't really feel mine. The surgeon cut the connection between my pregnancy and my baby when he cut into me.

> We made a life for the three of us as a family, but we did not seem close. Perhaps she was, and is, a very self-sufficient child.

> Physically my daughter has never felt part of me. My baby was never born.

Feelings like these often resolve themselves with time, and with the steps you can take, described in Chapter 8, to help yourself to come to terms with your caesarean experience. If, however, you feel that your childbirth experience is having a long-term deleterious effect on your relationship with your child, it would be wise to seek professional help. Your GP may be able to refer you to a counsellor, psychologist or family therapist. Other sources of help are listed in the useful addresses section on pages 237-8.

A CHILD'S-EYE VIEW

So far I have tended to look at the caesarean experience solely from the perspective of the mother, but what of the child's perspective? How do babies feel when they are born by caesarean? What are the effects of caesarean birth on children as they grow up? Does it influence the type of people they become? And what can we, as parents, do to help our children to see their birth and themselves in a positive light? There are, as yet, no definitive answers to such questions, given our present state of knowledge. But it is important to consider these issues, for without such consideration this account of the caesarean experience would be incomplete.

There is no way that we can ever really know how a baby feels during birth, but many women try to imagine how their baby must have felt. Some mothers whose babies are born by caesarean fear that the abrupt and unexpected transition from the warmth and security of the uterus to the cold, noisy and bright world outside is distressing for a baby. Others imagine that the experience of caesarean delivery is easier for a baby than vaginal delivery, with its seemingly unending contractions and the sometimes difficult journey down the birth canal. But what seems likely is that being born by caesarean is, in some ways, different from being born vaginally. And as the mother's experience of caesarean birth differs depending on the circumstances in which it is carried out, so too does the baby's experience. A caesarean carried out before the onset of labour is likely to be experienced differently by the baby than a caesarean performed after labour has begun. The infant's experience may also depend on whether he suffered from fetal distress prior to the caesarean, how easily he began breathing after the birth and whether general or regional anaesthesia was used.

Jane Butterfield English has written a fascinating book entitled *Different Doorway: Adventures of a Caesarean Born* which can provide some initial insights into how it feels to be born by caesarean.[37] She describes how she spent ten years exploring — through dreams and artwork, meditation, by re-living her own birth and by talking to others who were born by caesarean — what it means to be caesarean born, and the influence her birth had on her identity, her relationships and her life. She believes that the circumstances of our birth have a powerful influence on the way we see the world, and that caesarean birth can have negative but also positive and liberating effects on those who entered the world in this way.

English herself was born by caesarean before the onset of labour and describes vividly the feeling of being born so quickly, without the physical stimulation of contractions that usually presages the transition into the outside world, and the feeling of being undefended against the onslaught of new sensation at birth. She relates this to her subsequent feelings of being intruded upon and her tendency to push people away. Yet she also sees in herself a tendency to feel merged with everything, and to take on the emotions of those around her — something she speculates may result from being a non-labour caesarean since babies learn their first lessons about boundaries and separateness through their mother's labour. She also attributes her dependence on others and her sense of waiting to be rescued, to her birth by caesarean.

But there are other, positive aspects to being born by caesarean. To be cared for and nourished by a whole team of people at birth can be a positive experience which gives those born in this way a feeling of trust in the world at large, a sense that everything will be all right. English also sees in caesarean-born people the ability to take huge leaps with the help of others, and great skills at mobilising the resources of teams of people. She also suggests that, as a result of the patterns they learned at birth, those born vaginally often have a sense that life is a struggle, that change is slow and difficult and requires a lot of effort, whereas the caesarean born have a sense of limitlessness, that anything is possible, and can help others to see that there do not always have to be barriers.

Whilst English does not claim that all caesarean-born people will share these traits, as every caesarean birth is different and since birth is just one experience that shapes the type of people we become, she has provided a rough preliminary map that can be used as a starting point in understanding how people may feel about being born by caesarean.

One thing that can undoubtedly influence the way children feel about being caesarean born is the way we talk to them about birth in general and about their birth in particular. At first sight it might seem that explaining caesarean birth to a child is easier than describing vaginal birth, but this is not always the case. It is important for your child to know that she was born by caesarean, but also that not all babies come out this way, that most babies are born vaginally.

This will inevitably lead to questions about why his birth was different. It is not always easy to explain this in a way in which very young children can understand — my son was not yet 3 when he asked me, 'How did you take me out of your tummy?' and in a way that minimises children's tendencies to blame themselves for events. Nancy Cohen and Lois Estner point out that if you tell your child that he was born by caesarean because he was so 'big and strong' that he could not fit through the birth canal, the child may believe that he alone was responsible for his mother's surgery.[38] It may be best to tell your child simply that he was born by caesarean because both you and the doctors felt that this would be the safest way for him to be born. It may also be helpful to tell your child which of his friends were born by caesarean (many of us could compile quite a list!) so that he realises that, whilst caesarean birth is not the usual way for babies to be born, many babies are born this way and he is certainly not alone.

Children's questions about their birth are not mere intellectual curiosity — knowing the story of their birth helps them to learn about themselves and their place in the family and in the world. It is a story that your child may want to hear many times. Even if your experience of caesarean birth was a very difficult one, there will invariably be some positive aspects to it, and when talking to your child it is important to focus on these. Sheila Kitzinger and Celia Kitzinger describe how a woman who has had a caesarean with regional anaesthesia may talk to her child about how she decided to have a painkiller that did not send her to sleep so that she could be there to welcome her baby, how daddy was there, how he helped, how everyone worked together and how she felt when she saw her child being lifted into the world and when she first held her in her arms. Similarly, a caesarean mother who had general anaesthesia may explain to her child that a sudden decision had to be made to carry out a caesarean and that she had to be put to sleep for a short while, how daddy cuddled and cared for him until she woke up, how she felt when she first saw her baby and about all the people who helped her to have the baby safely and later cared for them both.[39]

If your own experience of caesarean childbirth was a positive one, then to speak positively about the birth to your child is relatively straightforward:

> My children have been brought up to see childbirth as a happy, normal event — in which medical help is occasionally needed. They have seen my scar and heard the stories of their births.

My son likes to joke that he couldn't find his way out!

Messages about your child's birth may also be conveyed indirectly. There is a children's book entitled *Are You My Mother?*[40] which I enjoy reading to my son and which he likes to hear over and over again. It is the story of baby bird who hatches whilst his mother is away from the nest looking for food for her soon-to-hatch chicks. The baby bird leaves his nest and has many adventures looking for his mother, until he is put safely back in his nest just as she returns. He knows immediately that she is his mother, and the book ends with a picture of the baby bird nestled under his mother's wing. I later realised that the attraction this book held for both myself and my son may have been because the story is a powerful analogy of our experience at his birth (a caesarean under general anaesthesia).

One reason why it is not always easy to talk about caesarean birth to our children is that it is, for some, a very emotionally-laden subject. If your own experience was very distressing you may find yourself avoiding the topic with your child, or her questions about her birth may leave you in a stunned silence, not knowing what to say or where to begin. Your child may then sense your unease and begin to feel negative about her birth and perhaps even herself. This is all the more reason for you to begin the sometimes difficult, but often necessary, process of coming to terms with the caesarean experience — a process which is discussed in Chapter 8.

Child psychologist Bruno Bettelheim points out how important it is that, when parents discuss difficult experiences from their own past with their children, they do so with sensitivity and an awareness of the child's perspective.[41] He describes the potential negative effects of not talking to children about a distressing part of your life — that children may interpret the silence as a deliberate exclusion and may conclude that they are incompetent or unworthy of receiving your confidences.

But Bettelheim also points out the dangers that can arise when parents do share difficult experiences with their children. The child may believe that his mother has chosen to tell him about her difficult experience as a punishment for some imagined misdemeanour. He may conclude that under no circumstances must he give his parents any more reason to suffer, or he may feel he has an obligation to make up for the past by giving his parents only pleasure. All this becomes even more complicated when the difficult experience in question is the child's own birth. But if it is handled with care and sensitivity, then sharing with your child, particularly an older child, some of the painful emotions that arose from his birth can enrich your relationship and bring you closer together. For example, April Altman recounts a conversation she had with her caesarean-born daughter when she was expecting her third child and planning to have a normal delivery at home. She writes:

> Rivka, my oldest child, said to me 'Why can't you have the baby in hospital like you did with me ?' I think she was feeling that her birth was wrong, that she had done something wrong. At first I wanted her to feel all right about herself and her birth, so I told her that the cesarean wasn't so bad. But then I realized it was bad, and I didn't want her to grow up thinking that she should have her babies by cesarean. But I wanted her to know that the birth wasn't her fault. I said to her 'The cesarean was very upsetting. But the doctor didn't know that it was OK to deliver you vaginally. Both the doctor and I thought that this was the best thing at the time for you because we didn't know any better.' I let her know that I was very happy when she was born, that I could hold her and love her, but it wasn't the way I wanted the birth. Afterwards she seemed to feel better.[42]

7 Partners' Perspectives

There is a third person who, along with the mother and the baby, is intimately involved in the caesarean experience, and that is your partner. A partner is an adult that a woman feels close to and chooses to have with her during labour, during the birth or soon afterwards — it may be a friend or your mother, for example. In most instances, it is the baby's father, but most of what I write in this chapter also applies to other types of partner.

When a woman gives birth by caesarean it can be a profound and moving experience for her partner, but just as each caesarean mother's experience is unique, so too are the experiences and feelings of partners. Some look back on the birth as being the happiest moment of their life; for others it is an event about which they have very mixed emotions; and for some it is a highly distressing experience. And yet the partner's perspectives are rarely discussed, either in day-to-day life or in accounts of caesarean childbirth. Consequently, partners may feel at a loss to describe the powerful and complex emotions that caesarean birth can evoke. One woman who took part in my research wrote that her partner could not answer my question about his feelings during the birth because he just could not put into words how he felt.

A FATHER'S PLACE

Thirty years ago the corridor outside the labour ward was seen as the appropriate place for a father at the birth of his child. But nowadays a father's place is seen as at the mother's side — at least for vaginal births. It is only in recent years that it has become common practice for fathers to be present at caesareans carried out under regional anaesthetic. And although a handful of consultants are willing to allow partners to be present when a caesarean is performed under general anaesthetic, most obstetricians feel that a father's place is most definitely not at the mother's side when the birth is a general anaesthetic caesarean.

In my research less than 3 per cent of partners were present when general anaesthesia was used, whereas 88 per cent of partners were at the birth when the caesarean was carried out with regional anaesthesia. To many caesarean parents this disparity seems baffling and illogical:

> I felt that my husband was shut out. I couldn't understand why he couldn't stay for the birth as they were willing to let him stay if I was awake, so why not when I was asleep?

A perhaps surprisingly large number of parents would like the baby's father to be present at caesarean births with general anaesthesia. In my own research, for more than half of all couples whose partner was excluded from a general anaesthetic caesarean, both parents wanted the father to be present.[1] Other researchers have also found that many couples would like the father to be present in such circumstances and feel disappointed and angry when he is excluded.[2] In some hospitals, partners are given the option of watching the birth through the viewing window of the operating theatre — a compromise solution that is much appreciated by some, but which others see as a frustrating half-way house.

The Caesarean Support Network recently carried out an informal survey of consultant obstetricians' views about fathers being present at general anaesthetic caesareans.[3] Only one of the consultants contacted was willing to allow partners to be present. The overwhelming majority took the view that it would be most inappropriate for partners to be permitted to witness caesarean births under general anaesthetic.

Some obstetricians felt that when general anaesthesia is used, the father, being an observer with no clearly defined role (unlike in epidural caesareans where the father has a specific and active role in supporting the mother), might 'get in the way' and hinder the team carrying out the caesarean. Some commented that a partner would be a liability in the operating theatre should he faint or feel ill, but there is little reason why a partner should be any more likely to faint at a caesarean under general anaesthetic than one with regional anaesthesia.

Others felt that it would be very distressing for a father to see the mother unconscious and intubated (that is, with a tracheal tube in place). Whilst the process of intubation may well be unpleasant to witness, there is no reason why partners could not wait outside until intubation is complete. It seems unlikely that all partners would find the sight of a person unconscious and already intubated unduly distressing since this is a relatively commonplace sight in television dramas and documentaries. Surely, then, this should be a matter for individual couples to decide rather than banning all partners from the operating theatre for general anaesthetic caesareans.

Some obstetricians pointed out that caesareans carried out under general anaesthetic are more likely to be emergency caesareans, and to have a partner present in such a situation would be off-putting for the operating team, and would be upsetting for the partner. But by no means all general anaesthetic caesareans are emergencies, and to apply a blanket ruling on this basis does not seem warranted. Others pointed out that serious complications can occur during caesareans, and it would be very distressing for a partner to witness this. But this is not a particularly strong argument for excluding partners from general anaesthetic caesareans since things can also occasionally go seriously wrong during caesareans under regional anaesthesia and during vaginal births. Also, whilst it is evident that witnessing a caesarean where serious complications arise is highly traumatic, it can be argued that this is, in itself, no justification for excluding partners. For example, obstetrician Peter Huntingford writes: 'In my experience no anticipated complications or even tragedy at the birth justifies the exclusion of the father. Sooner or later the truth has to be known and fantasies are usually worse than reality. In the end it is usually easier to accept and come to terms with what happens if you have been a witness to events as they unfold, rather than if bad news is conveyed to you by a stranger afterwards. The sharing of sorrow and pain is just as important as the sharing of happiness.'[4]

Many obstetricians justified their different rules for epidural and general anaesthetic caesareans on the grounds that when regional anaesthesia is used the partner has a very important role in supporting the caesarean mother during the birth, support which he cannot provide when the woman is unconscious. They also pointed out that with regional anaesthesia the birth is a shared experience for the parents, an experience that cannot be shared when general anaesthesia is used. But, although this is true, there are a number of important ways in which a partner's presence can help the caesarean couple and make the whole experience more positive.

When a partner is present he can be there to greet the baby as soon after the birth as possible and to welcome him into the world. For as one caesarean mother wrote in response to the Caesarean Support Network's survey on this matter, 'Many caesarean mothers have strong feelings of guilt about "not being there" and it would offer some consolation to them to know that, at least, their partner had been there.'[5]

Having your partner present can also be very helpful because he will be able to recount the birth to you, making it seem more real, and helping you to create an image of your child's birth:

> My husband did ask if he could stay, but he had to wait outside, and I do feel that had he been present then I could at least have felt that one of us was there to see him born, and I could have questioned him about it afterwards.

> My sister had been with me during my labour (I am a single parent) but was not allowed into the operating theatre. I feel if she had been at least she could have said, 'I saw them lift him from your womb covered in blood.'

Of course it is possible for a member of the medical team present at the caesarean to describe and recount the birth — something which many of us would greatly appreciate — but unfortunately this is something that is rarely offered at present. Also, as Peter Huntingford rightly points out, a partner can describe the birth with details that a professional attendant might consider trivial and this can do a lot to make up for what the baby's mother missed.[6]

It is also important to remember that a caesarean is not like any other operation — it is a birth. The birth of a baby is one of life's most momentous events, whatever the mode of delivery. When caesarean parents say that they would like the partner to be present at the birth, this is not some kind of voyeurism; it is the natural desire to witness that most precious moment when a child is born.

It is apparent that a partner's presence can have a number of beneficial effects. Indeed, research indicates that couples tend to feel more positive about the whole caesarean experience when partners are present at the delivery.[7] The benefits of partner presence must be weighed against potential disadvantages (for example, some partners would undoubtedly find it a distressing experience), so that you and your partner can come to the decision that is right for you as a couple. For doctors to make this decision on behalf of caesarean parents is both paternalistic and ultimately unhelpful.

Partners are usually welcome when caesareans are carried out with regional anaesthesia, but this is not always the case. One woman in my research was told that her partner could not be present because the operating theatre was too small, and another was told simply that her consultant did not allow partners into the operating theatre whatever the type of anaesthesia used. In some hospitals, partners are encouraged to attend elective epidural caesareans, but are not permitted to stay for unplanned epidural caesarean births. Sometimes the whole question is evaded:

> I wanted an epidural so I would be awake. I wanted Gary to be there to witness the birth, but I was never actually asked and he never actually pushed himself to be there.

It is important to recognise, however, that not all partners will want to be present, even at caesareans with regional anaesthesia, and their wishes should also be respected. No one should feel pressured to be present at a caesarean birth (or any other kind of birth, for that matter). You and your partner may have valid reasons for not wanting him to be there at the birth:

He was with me throughout my labour, but not for the caesarean. He couldn't stand seeing me being 'cut up'.

Some couples will know straight away that they would like the baby's father to be present at a caesarean birth; other couples have little difficulty in deciding that this is not something for them. But for some the decision can be very difficult. One partner described it like this:

It was a bit like being given the opportunity to parachute out of an aeroplane — something you felt you shouldn't pass up, since you had the opportunity, but that you really, really didn't want to do.

If you and your partner decide that you would like your partner to be present at the caesarean birth, but your consultant is unwilling to allow this, there are a number of steps you can take. You can speak to your consultant about the matter — consultants do occasionally relent after an initial refusal. Consultants differ in their views and it may be possible to change to another consultant or to another hospital where your wishes can be accommodated — this can be arranged through your GP. It can, however, be quite a battle. In 1989, the Caesarean Support Network in Britain detailed one man's campaign to be present should his wife need a caesarean under general anaesthetic.[8] After his request to be present was refused he asked his MP to take up the matter on his behalf, but the Government's position appears to be that the question of whether partners are present at general anaesthetic caesareans is a matter for the clinical judgement of the doctor concerned. He pressed on and arranged a further meeting with the consultant, a representative of the local health authority and a hospital administrator. Following this meeting, on the very day his wife went into labour, he received written confirmation that he could be present should the need for a general anaesthetic caesarean arise.

BEING THERE

What is it like to be present at a birth that is also an operation? It is not possible to provide any definitive answers to this question since all individuals react differently and since no two caesarean births are identical. But partners' emotions at this time often follow a common pattern. The majority of partners report feeling both apprehensive and happy during the birth.[9] They may be frightened that something might go wrong, concerned for the well-being of the mother and often for the safety of the baby as well. They sometimes worry about how they are going to cope in this unusual and potentially stressful situation. But the moment when the baby is lifted out is typically one of marvel and joy — a moment that most partners will treasure for years to come. One father wrote:

> I was very worried during the ten minutes that they prepped Dawn. I changed into the theatre gown as fast as possible then spent five minutes worrying that they had started without me. I was wondering what was happening and I did not want to miss the birth as she had chosen an epidural so I could be there. I was impressed with the speed of the operation and I felt totally elated when they handed the baby to me.

A substantial minority of partners apparently had no fears during the caesarean and reported feeling only joy and elation:

> He felt part of his son's birth and very proud to have been my strength and comfort. Also, he was the first to hold our son, not as usual the mother first. In fact, he nearly fell off his stool craning his neck to take in every detail of the baby while they cleaned him up.

Just a handful of the partners in my research reported that their predominant emotion during the birth was one of fear.

When regional anaesthesia is used partners have a crucial role to play in providing emotional support:

> Simon stayed with me throughout and was a great comfort to me. I was shaking uncontrollably, I suppose due to the drugs

and fear, and to have Simon talking softly to me and stroking my arms and hair was very reassuring.

Partners are often concerned about the question of where to look, and whether or not to watch the operation itself. In most cases, the father sits at the mother's side, his attention focused on her rather than the operation, and once the baby is born both parents turn all their attention to the newborn:

I need not have worried about the gore, because it was perfectly possible to keep behind the screens, and anyway there was plenty to do distracting my wife and assisting with breathing.

However, a minority of partners do watch the operation itself:

He amazed himself — and me — by coping with being there, and by deliberately watching the birth when he didn't need to with the screen up. Normally he only has to see a cut finger or hear someone talk of blood or anything slightly gory to come over all funny and have to look away! He says he wouldn't have missed it for anything.

The experiences above relate to partners who were present at caesareans with regional anaesthesia. Because it is so unusual, at present, for partners to be there when caesareans are carried out under general anaesthetic, we know very little about this experience, and whether the type of anaesthesia alters the way partners feel during a caesarean birth. When general anaesthesia is used, the vast majority of partners find themselves in the corridor or a room outside the operating theatre.

PACING THE CORRIDOR

My husband feels cheated. He sat through two labours only to be pushed out to pace the corridor and worry. We couldn't share such an important event.

Feelings like these are quite common when a caesarean is carried out under general anaesthetic and partners are excluded. Some couples find it very distressing to be separated at this time, particularly after sharing the intimate closeness that many experience during labour.

Waiting for news that the baby has been born and that all is well can be a very difficult time for partners. This wait is usually around ten minutes, but according to one father it can seem more like ten hours. The predominant emotions at this time tend to be fear and concern for the mother and baby, and a sense of powerlessness and helplessness. These feelings are exacerbated when there is a delay, and although delays do not necessarily mean that a problem has arisen, this is the conclusion that partners often draw.

A number of partners also feel a sense of disappointment that they were unable to witness the birth and to share this precious moment with the baby's mother. Nowadays, it is the norm for men to be present during childbirth, and one of the questions most frequently asked of new fathers is 'Were you there at the birth?' This can leave caesarean fathers who did not witness the birth with a sense of having missed out:

My husband was bitterly disappointed that he couldn't see our son born, he had been really looking forward to it.

Some caesarean mothers feel this sense of disappointment on behalf of their partners and blame themselves for his exclusion:

I feel so guilty that my husband couldn't be there.

The first thing that I felt after the initial 'Is she all right?' was that I had let my husband down. For weeks his friends had been ribbing him with tales of their children's births, and I felt he had been cheated of the experience.

Providing all is well, the new baby is brought out to his father only minutes after the birth. As he meets and greets his newborn the emotions he felt during the wait are replaced by feelings of joy and awe, as he holds him in his arms for the first time —

something that one caesarean father described as an 'emotional flip-flop':[10]

> Once the baby had been checked over he was taken swiftly to my waiting husband who immediately broke down in tears — it was a mixture of sheer relief and joy at the same time.

For some partners, however, these positive emotions are mixed with worry and concern for the mother:

> He says that when he was given our baby he was quite happy to hold her, but what he really wanted to do was to be back with me.

It is very important that the baby is handed to his father as soon as possible after the birth, for this is something that not only fathers but also mothers greatly appreciate:

> My husband held our daughter when she was four minutes old which I thought was absolutely wonderful and completely made up for me not seeing her straight away.

Occasionally, however, a mother may feel jealous of her partner's time with the new baby:

> I felt that my husband and son formed part of a family from which I was excluded and I was terribly jealous of them and their relationship.

FATHER AND CHILD

Some fathers worry that the fact that they were not present at the birth may have a deleterious effect on their subsequent relationship with their child. But although there is a widespread belief that a special bond is created when a man witnesses the birth of his child, there is very little research evidence to support this view.[11] As I pointed out in Chapter 6, bonding is a long-term process, not something that happens instantaneously at birth.

Some parents feel that a stronger bond is formed between father and child when the birth is by caesarean:

> I think in some respects my husband is as close to our son as he is because of the role he had to play in welcoming him on his own.

Also, because we are often limited in what we can do for our babies after having a caesarean, our partners may find themselves more involved in caring for the baby, dressing her and changing nappies, than they might otherwise have been, and this can lay the foundation for a close relationship between father and child. Indeed, research confirms that caesarean fathers tend to be more actively involved in childcare than other fathers, in the early weeks and months at least. [12]

There may occasionally be problems in the relationship between father and child if the father blames the child for the caesarean, but this is rare. In most cases, caesarean fathers feel as close, or sometimes closer, to their infants than fathers whose children were born vaginally.

MIXED EMOTIONS

Many caesarean fathers have mixed emotions about the birth. When the decision to carry out a caesarean is made, some partners feel upset or angry, but others feel a great sense of relief, particularly if the decision follows a long and difficult labour — relief that the labour will soon be over and that the baby will at last be born. If the baby is in distress partners may fear for the baby's life. During the birth itself there are the mixed emotions of worry and concern, then joy and elation described above. There are also the numerous feelings relating to being present or not being present at the birth.

In the weeks and months that follow the birth partners may experience other emotions. Some feel positive about the whole birth experience and remember it as either a peak moment in their life or a much needed life-saving measure for which they are extremely grateful. But some partners continue to feel a sense of loss that they were not present at the birth. Others experience a sense of guilt that they, unlike the mother, came through the experience physically unscathed. Caesarean father Paul Cohen wrote:

> I felt guilty for being downstairs while my wife was on the operating table. It should have been me, I thought. [13]

Others report feelings of failure, that they did not do all that they could have done to help their partner have a vaginal delivery and avoid a caesarean:

> My husband had been as excited as me to start with, but he was devastated by the eventual birth. He felt he should have done more for me, though he doesn't know what. In the end he just felt helpless.

The way partners feel depends to a large extent on the circumstances of the birth — whether it was a first or subsequent caesarean; on the type of anaesthesia used; whether it was an elective or emergency caesarean; on whether or not they were present; and on whether it was a medically straightforward caesarean or whether complications arose.

But like caesarean mothers, the way fathers feel will also depend on less tangible psycho-social factors such as their expectations about the birth, the extent to which they are involved and informed in decisions, how necessary they perceived the caesarean to be and how supported they felt during the whole experience.

When partners hold high expectations about the birth and envisage a normal vaginal delivery, they may find it difficult if the birth turns out to be a caesarean:

> My husband tried to keep positive for me, but he was disappointed. Having been to NCT classes we were both looking forward to the birth experience. All around us couples were experiencing birth normally — it was very hard for him.

Equally, when partners are not involved in or even informed of decisions taken during labour, or receive no explanation as to why a caesarean is necessary, then they are less likely to feel happy about the birth:

> My husband was very upset as not a lot had been explained to him during labour and the section.

Partners can be left feeling both powerless and angry if they perceive that the caesarean was not entirely necessary or if they feel that a caesarean could have been avoided had the labour been managed differently.

They also need a certain level of support if they are to feel positive about the birth. A partner who is present at the birth may need some reassurance and should be made to feel that he is welcome. Partners who are not present usually find it helpful if someone can wait with them, rather than being left alone at what may be a distressing time. The time when a father meets and greets his newborn baby is also very important. Insensitive treatment at this time can leave partners feeling angry and let down:

> Outside the theatre the nurse shouted to Andy, 'You have a little boy.' She handed him to him and he held him for a little while, whilst she got a bit of paperwork done. Then she took him from him and said, 'That's enough now, get back to the waiting room.' He was very annoyed.

Although I have tended to focus on negative experiences in this section, I do not want to give the impression that caesarean birth is always or inevitably a difficult experience for partners. It can be a really positive experience, as the following account shows:

> I was surprised and pleased that it was taken for granted that I would be present. The actual operation amazed me with its speed, climaxing four days of labour with ten minutes of fear (on my part), before our baby was in our arms, and twenty minutes of joyful tears while the stitches were made, before we left the theatre. I was sorry not to see our baby appear, but was more than compensated by the look on Susannah's face as she watched the scene reflected in the surgeon's glasses. The

following hours were filled with pride, at being a father and at seeing my Susannah walking about only a few hours after the operation, a feeling that is just as strong as I write this seven months later. As far as caesareans are concerned, I have no bad feelings about the operation or its after-effects — faced with no alternative we were quite comfortable with the operation. The really joyous thing about giving birth is not the method, but the result and, provided the parents are treated as participants in the operation rather than subjects of it, only positive feelings can ensue.

YOUR RELATIONSHIP AFTER A CAESAREAN

Caesarean childbirth, like any major life-event, can have lasting repercussions on your relationship as a couple. If the experience was a good one then you may well feel closer to each other as a result. But where there is a mismatch between the way you and your partner feel about the caesarean this can cause some strain in your relationship. Also, if you both found the experience a distressing one, this has the potential to cause a rift in your relationship unless you are able to cope with and accept the emotional pain each of you is feeling, and find ways of helping each other to come to terms with the experience.

Some partners find it difficult to understand why a woman might feel upset about giving birth by caesarean:

I think that he doesn't really understand. As far as he is concerned the scar is healed, therefore I'm better.

Even when partners are understanding, it can still be very difficult for them to provide the emotional support that women need after a distressing caesarean experience. For example, Paul Cohen, whose wife perceived her caesarean as unnecessary, wrote:

I felt scared for her emotional well-being, and frustrated that I could not make it all better for her. I vacillated between wanting to support her concerns about the birth, and being impatient with her prolonged depression.[14]

The effects of caesarean birth can also extend to your sex-life. Sometimes women feel reluctant to resume love-making after a caesarean because of its physical effects, tiredness or sometimes because they dislike their scar or feel less feminine. But men can also feel reluctant:

> I was concerned that my husband seemed very inhibited about any sexual contact. Over a long period we managed to talk about our feelings and it emerged that he felt hypersensitive towards me. It seems that watching the operation and 'seeing inside me' had a profound effect on him and he was extremely worried about hurting me or, I suppose, my getting pregnant again.

Similarly, Nancy Cohen and Lois Estner cite the example of a doctor who had visions of his wife's belly ripping open when they made love.[15] Some men also feel very wary about having any more children:

> My husband was, I think, terrified by the whole experience and although we'd always said we only wanted to have two children, I am sure that the fact of Rosie's mode of birth had a great influence over his (and my) decision to have a vasectomy when she was ten months old.

There are a number of ways in which you can help each other after a difficult caesarean. Perhaps the most important thing is to talk to each other and to listen to and acknowledge what each of you has experienced. Your perspectives on the birth may well differ, but this does not mean that one of you is right and the other is wrong. A father may have difficulty sharing his feelings about the caesarean, for he may feel that it is self-indulgent to speak of his own emotional pain when it was not he himself who underwent the caesarean. But his pain is no less real, and also needs to be shared and acknowledged. Fathers also have an important role to play in helping caesarean mothers come to terms with what has happened to them. Many women will want to know that their partner understands their disappointment at not giving birth vaginally:

> I am lucky in having a husband who tried to understand my feelings and did not fob me off with 'well the main thing is that you and the baby are all right'.

Other women need their partner to acknowledge that the way they brought their child into the world was valid and courageous:

> Through it all my husband has been wonderful. He's always told me that it doesn't matter how our baby came into the world and that it makes him more precious because we had to struggle to keep him alive, and that I was braver than others who constantly whine on about how bad their birth was because all my pain came afterwards.

Ultimately, a positive caesarean experience, or one which couples share and come to terms with together, can strengthen relationships and bring about a mutual closeness. For instance, the father of four caesarean children was able to write:

> The scars, which now spell the initial letter of my nickname upside down, are still fading, but are still fun to trace, a private sign of our adventures together.

8 Coming to Terms

This chapter takes us into the fourth and final stage that follows caesarean birth — after shock, denial, sadness and anger, the stage when we begin to accept and come to terms with the whole experience. Because the process of emotional healing is unique to each individual, it is not appropriate to prescribe a set method for coming to terms with a caesarean delivery. Indeed, if your caesarean experience was a good one there may be very little that you have to come to terms with. What I hope to provide are some suggestions that others have found helpful and which may be of help to you.

Coming to terms with a difficult caesarean is a long and gradual process: acceptance comes in degrees. As the months and years pass you may notice that the birth is less often in your thoughts; you no longer find it distressing to watch operations on television; you are able to listen to accounts of natural births without feeling upset about your own childbirth experience; as you re-read an account of your experiences that you wrote some time ago, you realise that you no longer feel that way, and are taken aback at the intensity of the emotional pain you felt at that time; and you feel ready to contemplate another pregnancy.

Time is a great healer, but often time alone will not ease your emotional pain. Several of the women in my research reported that they still had difficult feelings about their caesareans two, three or four years after the event:[1]

> My experience of a caesarean childbirth happened nearly four years ago, and even at this time I still feel cheated, disappointed, a failure, that life's unfair, that I could have tried harder.

One woman was still very upset about a caesarean birth that happened ten years ago. Yet there is generally little recognition of how long it might take to come to terms with a caesarean delivery. People seem to expect the emotional wound to heal as quickly as the physical one:

> After about six weeks or so, everyone seemed to think I shouldn't be upset any longer — that I should be grateful for having such a lovely baby. Well, I am grateful, and I love my baby very much, but still wish I could have given birth to him.

The process of coming to terms with a difficult caesarean birth is rarely straightforward, for such a birth can evoke a complicated mix of emotions. Having a caesarean may have been both the most happy time of your life when your baby entered the world but also one of the most traumatic experiences that has ever happened to you:

> There are so many emotions. The bad ones block the good ones.

To integrate and accept these positive and negative emotions is not always easy. Sometimes the most difficult part is letting yourself believe that it is all right to feel sad about the caesarean. In our culture, the emotional pain that follows an unhappy childbirth experience tends to be dismissed — a healthy mother and baby are seen as all that matters. We, too, may find ourselves disowning our distress. Several women in my research wrote, 'I know it's selfish, but . . .', as though it is improper to have any negative feelings relating to our babies' births. But it is possible to feel immense gratitude that your baby is alive and well, and yet at the same time to feel very sad that a caesarean was necessary. The two feelings are not contradictory, although this is often how it feels. Your sense of loss is real and important, not a sign of selfishness. Sad and angry feelings are normal and essential parts of the grieving process.

It can also be difficult when other caesarean mothers appear to have only positive feelings about their births. They may indeed have had good experiences, but this does not mean that you are wrong to have difficult feelings about your own experience, for no two caesareans are alike, and some are much harder to come to terms with than others:

I felt guilty because most other people I know who have had caesars seem happy with them.

Equally, other caesarean mothers may be very reticent about revealing how they really feel about their caesareans, particularly in casual conversation.

It is also important to realise that, if you are planning to have more children, you are unlikely to be able to 'put it all behind you', since the whole experience is often forced back into your mind and emotions during a subsequent pregnancy:

I thought I had almost come to terms with the operation despite my desire for a natural birth, but the prospect of a repeat performance has brought back all the doubts and anxieties which I associate with the management of the last labour, and the lack of regard shown to my previously expressed wishes.

Despite all the difficulties, it is well worth embarking on the process of coming to terms with your caesarean birth, for in doing so you may well emerge with a positive perspective on your caesarean, and will ultimately feel at peace with the whole experience.

TALKING IT THROUGH

Perhaps the most important thing that you can do to help yourself to come to terms with your caesarean is to talk about it — to put into words all the complex, contradictory and painful emotions that you feel. In doing so, your feelings will begin to make some sense, and will no longer seem to be constantly clamouring for your attention. Talking about how you feel may well be painful, but to experience these negative feelings, and to acknowledge them as legitimate emotions, is an important step towards emotional recovery:

It helped to say, 'I'm really upset about not giving birth normally even though I know I am lucky to have a healthy baby.'

We often feel a deep need to talk about our caesarean experiences. Yet we may feel very wary of speaking about how we really feel because we are afraid of becoming overwhelmed by our distress or because it hurts to re-open the emotional wound. We may find ourselves reeling off details of times, places and events surrounding the caesarean and yet not really touching upon how we felt about it. Sometimes, we are reluctant to talk simply because we feel that no one would be interested to hear what we have to say. As time passes, it may seem inappropriate to talk about something that happened months or even years ago. But the need to talk remains. One woman wrote more than a year after her daughter was born by caesarean:

> I would desperately like to talk to someone even now, as I could not cope with being pregnant again.

You are unlikely to want to talk to just anyone about how you feel. Indeed, to do so might even be counterproductive because the other person might respond inappropriately with a hurtful, insensitive or jokey comment, or quickly change the subject. Such responses are likely to leave us feeling more vulnerable, unheard and alone in our distress. When deciding who to talk to, choose carefully and test the water with a few tentative comments before launching into how you really feel.

You might want to begin by talking to yourself, going over the experience in your head and putting your feelings into words:

> I used to relive it and go through the conversations again that took place, and the things I had said and felt. Those feelings gradually wore off and now, six months later, I don't feel this need.

Writing down your feelings can also be a very potent way of laying some of your feelings to rest. You may find that this helps to stop the thoughts and feelings that may seem to revolve endlessly in your head. It is also a good way of expressing your feelings when there is apparently no one with whom you can talk about them, or when talking is still too painful. Expressing how you feel in one way or another is so important, since when we hold on to our feelings they remain with us and the process of coming to terms is delayed. One woman wrote to me three years after her son's caesarean birth:

> I have wanted to tell someone who was interested about my caesarean birth for so long I don't know where to begin.

Try to write down everything that you felt and feel, the good feelings and the bad ones, even the ones that seem silly or illogical. Do not worry if your account is very long, jumbled or contradictory — many are. Emotions are rarely straightforward. You might want to simply put your writings in an envelope and keep it somewhere safe. Or you may like someone to read them — your partner, a close friend or another caesarean mother.

The person to whom women most often turn when they feel ready to talk is their partner. A partner needs to be able to listen uncritically, with patience, and to accept and acknowledge your feelings. Whilst many women find their partners invaluable in this respect, some partners are unable to help:

> Most people's attitudes, including my husband's, is that it's over now, and that you should make the most of what you've got and not hanker after the impossible dream.

Some women find it helpful to share their feelings with their caesarean-born children. This requires care, honesty and sensitivity to the child's needs, as discussed in Chapter 6, but it is something from which both mother and child can benefit. For example, Nancy Cohen and Lois Estner describe how one caesarean mother, who felt particularly sad about the enforced separation from her baby daughter after the birth, shared her feelings with her daughter, now aged 8. She took her daughter in her arms and told her all the things that she had wanted to say to her when she was newly born.[2]

Friends can also be useful people to talk to. A close friend will be able to listen to your experiences and feelings without judging you or making light of all that has happened to you. But some friends may find it difficult to understand your concerns, particularly if they are not mothers, or if their childbirth experiences were very different from your own. For this reason, you may find it more helpful to speak to other caesarean mothers:

> In the months that followed Tom's birth I found it helpful to talk to others who had had caesarean births. Other people were interested to hear about my experience and it helped to talk about it and to feel I still achieved something — even though the community midwife's comment when she visited me afterwards was that childbirth obviously wasn't something I was good at!

> It wasn't until I joined — and helped to form — a caesarean support group, when my daughter was 4 months old, that I eventually realised my feelings weren't so unusual for a 'caesarean mum'.

There are a number of caesarean support groups throughout Britain (see pages 237–8 for addresses). Such groups can provide an opportunity to talk about your caesarean to others who have had similar experiences, emotional support, information and the chance to help others to come to terms with their caesarean experiences. Some groups are also involved in campaigning for changes that will help other caesarean mothers, creating something positive out of negative experiences:

> Because of the support, or lack of it, I received during and after the birth I started my own caesarean support group. Our aim is to improve information to caesarean mums before, in antenatal classes, and after the birth.

> I've now met other women who've had caesareans at the same hospital and I've found that many of them have had similar experiences regarding their postnatal care. I am now trying to turn some of my anger into energy for changing things for other caesarean mums.

Some women also value the opportunity to share their feelings with those involved in their medical care — their midwife, health visitor or GP. Unfortunately, this does not always happen:

At no time after the birth of my child did anyone connected with the hospital or my own doctor ever seem interested to hear how I felt about it. This, I feel, would have been of major importance.

However, when health professionals are able to sit and listen to caesarean mothers, even for a short while, this can be enormously helpful:

At home I was visited by one midwife who commented that it was a shame it had turned out this way. I can hardly describe the relief I felt that somebody had acknowledged my feelings.

My health visitor really did help me to pick up the pieces. Her support kept me going.

If you have had a difficult caesarean experience which has left you feeling distressed or depressed you may feel in need of some form of counselling. Some of the women in my research received counselling or psychotherapy and found it very helpful. Your GP may be able to refer you to a counsellor, a psychologist or a psychiatrist. Alternatively, there are a number of other counselling services available, and these are listed on pages 237-8.

Finally, it is important to be aware that it is not usually enough to talk about your experiences and feelings just once. If your experience was a difficult one, you may well need to talk it through several times, maybe with different people, since coming to terms with a caesarean birth is a long and gradual process that does not happen overnight.

MISSING PIECES

Psychologist Dyanne Affonso talked to new mothers two to three days after giving birth and found that the majority reported being unable to remember one or more event in their labour or delivery and were attempting to recall these events. This sometimes led to repeated questioning, preoccupation and recurrent dreams. Affonso calls the events that the women could not recall 'missing pieces' and speculates that finding these missing pieces is a vital part of the process of integrating and accepting the birth experience.[3] For the caesarean mother who has had general anaesthesia, it is not little pieces of the birth experience that are missing, but huge chunks:

> I still feel that an important part of our history is missing because none of us will remember Daniel's birth.

If your caesarean was carried out under general anaesthesia, you may find it very helpful if you are able to recover some of the missing parts of your birth experience. If your caesarean is very recent, you may be able to speak to someone at the birth who remembers it and can describe it to you. Some women find it useful to watch a video of a caesarean birth, for this helps them to create an image of their own child's birth (see page 237 for details of how to obtain videos of caesarean births). By talking to your partner you can form quite an accurate picture of what happened during the time when your partner was with the baby before you regained consciousness.

You might also find it helpful to visualise your baby's birth, either as the caesarean that it was or the way you would like it to have been. This visualisation can help to provide a sense of closure to an experience that may otherwise feel somewhat unfinished:

> In the days immediately following the caesarean I kept wishing I could have the time back, to try again, rather like when you fail an examination. I even went as far as to take my tiny daughter, once we were home, and put her between my legs, pretending that I was giving birth.

Whatever type of anaesthesia you had, you may find that you cannot clearly recall parts of your labour or events that occurred prior to the caesarean, or you may have difficulty remembering things that happened during your hospital stay. You may be able to piece together much of what happened by talking with your partner. Your hospital notes may also help you to work out exactly what happened to you, and when. Your notes will usually be left at the end of your bed while you are in hospital and there is no reason why you should not read them. Women are sometimes given their notes to look after when they are discharged from hospital and still under the care of the community midwife and this is another opportunity for you to read them. At a later date, you could write to the hospital asking for a copy of your notes — some hospitals are willing to provide such a thing.

You may feel that you are missing information about the reason for your caesarean, about the nature of and reasons for any complications you suffered, or about the likely management of future births. Such information is often vital if you are to come to terms with the birth. You are entitled to explanations about your caesarean, even if it took place several years ago. There is now growing recognition that explanations are an essential part of good medical care. If you did not receive an adequate explanation of why your caesarean was necessary, why some complication arose or what will happen in future deliveries, do ask before you leave hospital, and keep on asking until such explanations are forthcoming. You have another opportunity to ask these questions at your six-week check-up. After that, if you still have unanswered questions about your caesarean, you could ask your GP. He or she may well be able to answer your questions, since he or she will have received a summary of your hospital notes. If your GP does not have the information you require, he or she may be willing to refer you back to your consultant. Alternatively you could write to your consultant directly:

I was tormented by the thought that the caesarean was my own fault, and that I hadn't coped where others had. And I was angry that no one had attempted to explain things. I eventually wrote to my consultant and listed all of my questions relating to my labour and experiences. I wanted personal answers from my notes — not a textbook reply. I didn't expect a reply, but a few weeks later received a very detailed reply, answering all of my points individually. I found out medically what had happened during labour, at every stage, why the staff had done things like adjusting the drip control, all the little details and the sequence of events were confirmed. The letter concluded inviting me to visit my consultant personally if I had any other queries. I accepted this offer as my last chance to resolve the matter completely. My consultant was extremely kind and considerate when I met him. My final few queries were answered and he put my mind completely at rest, assuring me that I was in no way to blame for the need to perform a caesarean.

CAUSE FOR COMPLAINT

If parts of the care you received before, during or after your caesarean were unsatisfactory, you may find that you have cause for complaint. If this is the case, airing your grievances with your consultant or making a formal complaint can be crucial in helping you to come to terms with your experience. If your complaint is dealt with as it should be, then you will receive an honest explanation of what happened and why, an acknowledgement that what you experienced was unsatisfactory and perhaps also an apology. By making your complaint you are also helping to ensure that what happened to you will not happen to others. The knowledge that something positive has come out of your negative experience can be very consoling. When complaints are handled in this way, women are able to feel that although their experience was unfortunate, the matter is now resolved, it is in the past, and that they can begin to look to the future:

> We made three formal complaints to the hospital by letter and we were invited to visit the senior midwifery officer and a hospital administrator. This was a turning point. We catalogued all the dozens of awful things that had happened and the nasty comments that had been made by nurses, as well as explaining that one sister had been kind, and I cried a lot. It felt as if a great weight had been lifted.

Although it can be enormously beneficial, both to the individual concerned and to those who might otherwise have received similarly unsatisfactory care had a complaint not been received, not all women who have cause for complaint will wish to make one. You may be worried about what effect making a complaint will have on the care you receive if you have your next baby at the same hospital. Your subsequent care should not be adversely affected, but this is nevertheless a real concern for some women. You may not feel that you have the emotional or physical resources to make a complaint at a time when you are recovering from surgery and busy caring for a new baby. You may also be wary of becoming involved in something that can be, although is certainly not always, a long and drawn out process, when you just want to forget the whole experience. Only you can decide if making a complaint is the best course of action for you in your particular circumstances.

It is also a sad fact that not all complaints are resolved in a helpful or beneficial manner. The complaints system has been criticised for being 'totally inadequate' from the patient's point of view:[4]

> I was so upset by the whole chaotic performance that I wrote and complained to the hospital and received a rather bland, blasé reply about 'hospital policy', 'full explanations given', 'sorry that explanations had not been clear enough or reassuring', etc., and suggesting that I contact a caesarean support group.

Unfortunately, it is not uncommon for caesarean mothers' complaints about the management of their labour, delivery or postnatal care to be seen as evidence of the emotional distress resulting from having a caesarean or postnatal depression. This viewpoint is patronising, often incorrect and misses the point. It can feel very frustrating to have valid complaints dismissed and negated in this way.

If you do decide to make a complaint, there is a useful chapter in Beverley Lawrence Beech's book *Who's Having Your Baby?* which describes how to make a formal complaint (or in serious circumstances, legal action) following unsatisfactory maternity care.[5] You may also find it helpful to contact your local Community Health Council or AIMS (the Association for Improvements in the Maternity Services) for advice and support (see pages 237–8).

FOCUSING ON THE POSITIVE

Whilst talking about, and acknowledging, the negative side of having a caesarean is often essential if you are to accept and come to terms with the experience, it can also be very helpful to focus on the positive aspects of caesarean childbirth, for as one caesarean mother pointed out 'in order to survive life we all need to interpret its mishaps in a positive way'.

There are a number of ways of seeing your caesarean in a positive light. First and foremost there is the baby:

> For me the birth was not the end of a nine month wait, it was the beginning of something far more important and, while it was certainly a day to remember, the days, weeks and months that have followed are far more important to me.

> As time went by the bad bits got better and the baby was the more important part. My love and our relationship grew and his birth mattered less.

> I reckon I'd go through it all again ten times over to have another little one as gorgeous as Tom.

The knowledge that the caesarean saved your baby's life, or your own, or that it helped to prevent your baby from suffering brain damage or handicap can also help you to feel positive about the birth:

> The thing that has made me feel positive about the experiences is that in 'days of old' I wouldn't have survived the first pregnancy, nor would my son, never mind the second. I am extremely grateful.

Many caesarean mothers also feel positive about the fact that their birth canal has remained undamaged. However, it is important to remember that not all caesarean mothers will emerge with an intact perineum, and not all vaginal births result in an episiotomy or tear. Sometimes, a caesarean is carried out after forceps have failed. It is also fairly common for a woman's sex-life to be affected temporarily by having a caesarean, as discussed in Chapters 4 and 5. Nevertheless, if you do avoid an episiotomy or tear, this is something to feel positive about:

> I have to be blunt, I'm rather glad that my 'bits' are still intact — people have told me that you're never the same again after giving birth.

You should also be able to feel proud of yourself for all that you have achieved, for having met the challenge of caesarean childbirth:

> I've come to feel quite proud of having two fairly major operations in less than two years and still being able to chase round after a toddler a fortnight after the birth. It's time caesarean mums were given a pat on the back.

> I feel positive now because I have triumphed over an extra difficult birth and established and continued breastfeeding.

Finally, you may also be able to feel positive about the fact that when you consented to have a caesarean this was a decision made out of love for your baby, a decision about which any mother should feel proud. As one caesarean mother advises:

> Don't, whatever you do, feel a failure. Your decision to agree to the caesarean is not a giving up, but a giving of life.

A NEW PERSPECTIVE

As time passes and you talk through your experience, piecing together all that happened to you, the difficult and distressing parts and the joyous bits, until it forms an integrated whole, you will find that your emotional pain begins to fade. You may still feel sad that you gave birth by caesarean, but this sadness is no longer overwhelming. As Claudia Panuthos and Catherine Romeo point out, acceptance is not necessarily a happy state, but is more accurately the end of a long search for peace.[6] You begin to see your caesarean as an experience that is in the past, something that you cannot change and that you can accept:

> I would say that I haven't and never will come to terms with the fact that I had to have caesareans. I can live with this now but truthfully I would wish that this hadn't been so.

Other things in your life become more important and the birth takes its place in the background rather than the foreground of your emotions:

> I don't think the feelings change — just slip into the background as day-to-day life continues.

If you became very depressed following your caesarean, this too can pass:

> Gradually the depression lifted like a cloud passing overhead. Instead of every day being black, there were only certain 'bad' days a week. These in turn grew less and less frequent, until one day I suddenly realised I had not had a bad day for weeks. It was only then that I felt that I had finally come out of a long, long tunnel inside which there was only a twilight world of pain, sorrow, drudgery and despair.

Your experience of caesarean birth begins to take on a new perspective:

> I still catch my breath at the sight of an operating theatre, or green cloths, or the huge mirrored light over the operating table, and representations of birth on television or in novels are so very different that I feel a pang of sadness. But now, eight years since my first, and two and a half years since my last caesarean, I can accept the difference, even feel proud of it, and the momentary pangs are part of one image of reality jostling with another.

Ultimately, it is possible to feel positive about, and grow from, even the most difficult of caesarean experiences:

I have now completed the journey from the negative to a positive viewpoint. I now understand fully the reasons why I had to be delivered of my baby by caesarean section. I have succeeded in finding my own answers and consequently I have learned a great deal about myself. The baby that arrived in such an unnatural manner has grown into my daughter. I shall always be very sad and regretful that her arrival should have been such a traumatic experience, but at least I have been able to gain from it, and can now see it as a positive base on which to build.

9   Next Time

ANOTHER BABY?

The question of when and whether to have another child is something that faces most parents at some point after the birth of a baby. Coming to a decision about this is sometimes difficult, regardless of the earlier birth experience, but for caesarean parents there are often some additional concerns.

You may wonder when you will be medically fit to become pregnant again. Traditionally, caesarean mothers have been advised to wait at least a year after the caesarean before conceiving again to ensure that the wound is fully healed. But our bodies heal very quickly and not all obstetricians feel that it is necessary to wait this long. Obstetrician John Hare, for example, recommends a minimum gap of six months between pregnancies for both caesarean and vaginally-delivered mothers.[1] But obviously circumstances vary from woman to woman and it is important to wait until you feel ready to embark upon another pregnancy. As one woman wrote:

> Having a caesarean did make me reconsider the age gap between my children. When many friends who had their first children with me were onto their second, I was just beginning to feel fit again and being pregnant was the last thing on my mind.

For many caesarean mothers it is not just a question of feeling physically ready for another pregnancy, but also of whether they are emotionally ready to become pregnant again. If your experience of caesarean childbirth was a difficult one, it may take quite a while before you feel able to consider having another baby because you are wary of repeating the experience:

It took over two and a half years before I began to feel I'd like another baby. The possibility of another section filled me with dread.

At the time of the caesarean and shortly afterwards I was absolutely sure — no more babies. Now fifteen months on I can still remember clearly the bad times, but the good times are numerous and I'm not saying 'no more babies', I'm saying 'I'm thinking about it'.

If your caesarean was a positive experience, you may be very keen to have another baby. But it is not just those with positive feelings about their caesareans who can feel a strong desire to become pregnant soon after the first birth. Women who felt that they had 'failed' by giving birth by caesarean may experience a deep longing for another baby, a baby that they could give birth to vaginally. As one caesarean mother wrote:

I would like the chance to get it right next time.

For some women this need to give birth vaginally can be overwhelming. Nancy Cohen and Lois Estner give the example of a woman who had four caesareans in quick succession, when each time she had hoped for a vaginal birth. After her fifth child was born vaginally, she wrote:

I am no longer preoccupied with childbearing. It is all worked through now, and it is all healed. [2]

Sometimes the desire for another baby is matched by the fear of another caesarean, which makes the decision to have another baby a very difficult one:

For the first couple of years after my daughter's birth I see-sawed emotionally between longing to have another child 'properly', and fearing another caesarean, and possibly another bout of postnatal depression.

Because feelings can and often do change it would probably be advisable not to make any final decisions until at least a year after the birth, if not longer:

> When our son was about four months old, my husband had a vasectomy as we decided that we didn't want to go through the experience again, but I regret that my husband had the operation as I would now like a second child and feel that, with advice and encouragement, I could have a normal delivery second time around. However, it is not to be.

Over a third of the women in my research reported that having a caesarean had made them reconsider the number of children they wanted to have.[3] Sometimes this was because they found the caesareans physically or emotionally taxing. But sometimes caesarean mothers consider limiting the size of their family as a result of medical advice. A few decades ago caesarean mothers were advised to have no more than two children. A little later the limit was put at three children. But at present, as a result of improvements in surgical techniques, many doctors now suggest four caesareans as the upper limit. Caesarean parents can sometimes feel a little resentful that this most important decision — how many children to have — may be taken out of their hands and decided by an obstetrician:

> After my fourth caesarean I was told it would be inadvisable to have any more. We had previously discussed this as a possibility with the surgeon. It took me quite a while to come to terms with 'them' making the decision for me. Although in fact neither of us particularly wanted another child, I felt something of the feeling that I ought to so as it would be up to me not them!

In fact, in general, there is no absolute limit on the number of caesareans you may have — one woman is reputed to have had seventeen![4] However, the operation does become very demanding, technically and surgically, after four or five caesareans.

Some obstetricians will recommend that a woman be sterilised at the time of her third or fourth caesarean. The advantages of this are that it saves you from being 'opened up' again, and means that you only need one dose of anaesthesia. However, a sterilisation operation is very minor and may even be carried out under local anaesthetic, so these arguments for carrying out a sterilisation at the same time as a caesarean are not particularly strong. Many would advise against sterilisation at this time because it is often a very emotional time and feelings can change, so it may be sensible to wait until a later date.

ANOTHER CAESAREAN?

Something that is uppermost in the minds of many caesarean mothers when they embark upon another pregnancy is whether or not they will give birth by caesarean this time. In fact, around half of all women who have had one caesarean will have their next child by caesarean. For some, the subsequent caesarean will be an elective one, planned in advance. For others, it will be unplanned and carried out after a trial of labour has 'failed'.

A trial of labour is when a woman goes into labour hoping for a vaginal delivery, the labour is watched carefully, and everything is ready should a caesarean become necessary. A trial of labour following a previous caesarean is technically called a 'trial of scar', but I have decided to avoid using this term for two reasons. Firstly, trial of labour is the term which women themselves tend to use, as do some obstetricians.[5] Secondly, when a trial ends in a caesarean this is invariably because the labour has 'failed', if, for example, the labour has become prolonged or the baby has become distressed. It is extremely rare for a trial to end because the scar has 'failed'.

The proportion of women who have a trial of labour after a previous caesarean varies enormously from consultant to consultant, from hospital to hospital, and from country to country. Vaginal birth after a caesarean (VBAC – pronounced '*vee-back*') has a long history in Europe and Australia, but this is not so in the USA. Despite the mass of medical evidence attesting to the relative safety of trials of labour and VBACs, American obstetricians have been, and largely still are, very reticent about allowing caesarean mothers to go into labour. In the late 1970s, around 98 per cent of caesarean mothers in the USA had elective repeat caesareans in subsequent pregnancies.[6] More recently, however, there has been a fall in the number of scheduled repeat caesareans, largely as a result of pressure from caesarean mothers themselves.

The question of whether an elective caesarean or a trial of labour is the best course of action for a particular individual is not always straightforward. Two obstetricians may have very different opinions. However, all the medical evidence indicates that, unless there is a recurrent reason for carrying out a caesarean, or unless a new reason arises in the present pregnancy, it is safer to opt for a trial of labour. Although there is a very small risk of the previous caesarean scar separating during a subsequent labour, it is a question of the balance of risks, and this minimal risk is outweighed by the greater risk to both mother and baby of carrying out a caesarean when a vaginal delivery may well be possible (the risks of caesarean childbirth are discussed in Chapter 2).[7]

The risks of having an emergency caesarean after a trial of labour are slightly higher than the risks of an elective caesarean, but it is important to remember that the majority of women who have a trial of labour will give birth vaginally. The vaginal delivery rate following trials of labour after a previous caesarean is around 80 per cent.[8] Vaginal birth is generally safer than an elective caesarean delivery, so the overall balance of risks favours a trial of labour.

Although the medical evidence is quite clear, obstetric opinion on this matter appears to differ widely. Some obstetricians will strongly recommend a trial of labour, some will leave the decision up to the woman herself and others will agree to a trial only in the most optimal of circumstances.

If you are given the choice about having a trial of labour or an elective caesarean, you may know that you would definitely like to go ahead with the labour, you may feel strongly that an elective caesarean is the right option for you or you may not find it easy at all to decide what is the best course of action:

> My consultant had given me the option of a caesarean or a natural birth and I had to make the decision myself. It was an extremely difficult decision to make.

The decision you make will inevitably be coloured by the way the choices are presented to you. If your doctor talks solely about the risks of scar separation but fails to mention the risks of a caesarean, and if you are given the impression that your chances of giving birth vaginally are low, then you may well opt for an elective caesarean; but you may make quite a different decision if you are told that you are more than likely to deliver vaginally and that, in medical terms, a trial of labour is the logical choice.

But the decision to have a trial of labour or an elective caesarean is much more than just a medical decision. Carol McClain has studied how women make this decision and found that social goals were as central to the decision process as was the women's assessment of the medical risks.[9] She found that women tended not to focus on the probabilities of the outcomes of each course of action, but instead constructed mental images of what they anticipated might happen based on their past childbirth experiences, and reinforced their decision by thinking solely about the benefits of the alternative they preferred and the hazards of the alternative they rejected.

There are a number of valid reasons why a woman might opt to have an elective caesarean. Of course, if there is a sound medical reason for having another caesarean, then an elective caesarean delivery will be safest for both you and your baby. Another consideration that is very important to many women is that by having an elective caesarean they will be able to have regional anaesthesia and so be awake to witness the birth, whereas if they opted for a trial of labour there is a chance that there would not be enough time to administer an epidural or spinal should the need for a caesarean arise. Although many women do have regional anaesthetic caesareans when a trial of labour has 'failed', this is not always possible if the baby is in distress and needs to be born very quickly.

Caesarean mothers whose previous experience of labour was distressing, or who had a very long or painful labour, may be very keen to have an elective caesarean to avoid repeating the experience, particularly if they feel that they may well end up with another caesarean anyway. You are also likely to be less tired, and perhaps to recover more quickly, after an elective caesarean than a caesarean carried out after a trial of labour. Some women do not want a trial of labour as they feel that it might be very difficult for them to cope with their subsequent feelings of failure should the trial end in a caesarean. Others choose to have an elective caesarean because it is very important for them to feel in control and to have a fair idea of what is going to happen:

> Having had a long labour and a section, I would much prefer an elective section rather than a labour, so I look forward to my next pregnancy and birth because I know what is going to happen and can plan for it.

Another advantage of having an elective caesarean is that, in most cases, you will know when your baby will arrive, which means it will be easier to make arrangements for the care of your other children while you are in hospital, and for help around the house when you come home. You may also take into consideration the fact that, if you have an elective caesarean, you will usually have the opportunity to meet the doctor and anaesthetist who will carry out the caesarean beforehand, to get to know them and ask any remaining questions you may have, something that may not be possible when a caesarean is carried out after a trial of labour.

There are also many good reasons for deciding to have a trial of labour. First and foremost, if there is no new or recurring reason why a caesarean might be necessary, then you have an excellent chance of giving birth vaginally, and vaginal birth is generally far less debilitating and more satisfying than a caesarean delivery and carries fewer risks. Even if the trial of labour ends with another caesarean, you may well feel happy that you opted for a trial because it proved that a caesarean was indeed necessary — something that often cannot be known in advance. Some women find labour itself an exciting, challenging and satisfying experience. You will also know that your baby was born when she was supposed to be, that she chose her own birthday.

What I have written so far may give the impression that the decision to carry out an elective caesarean or to go for a trial of labour is typically made prior to, or early in, pregnancy. Whilst decisions are sometimes made early on, what often happens is that a trial of labour is agreed to in principle early in pregnancy, but a final decision is not made until the last few weeks before the birth. If you have previously had a caesarean and are hoping to have a trial of labour, your consultant will probably carry out a careful assessment at around 36 or 37 weeks of pregnancy, by feeling your abdomen to ascertain the size and position of the baby. You may also be asked to have a scan or a pelvic x-ray. It can be difficult not knowing until late in pregnancy whether you will be having a trial of labour or an elective caesarean, but it does help if you are given clear information about the circumstances under which an elective caesarean would be recommended.

Some obstetricians believe that a trial of labour is the best course of action, even when the baby appears to be large or is not lying in an ideal position. To those who take this stance the baby's size and position are relatively immaterial. Other obstetricians are only concerned about this when the mother's pelvis is smaller than average; but some see the baby's size and position as crucial whatever the woman's pelvic measurements, and would advise against a trial of labour if it is anything but ideal. Finding out the views of your consultant early in pregnancy, or before you become pregnant, can help you to feel that you have a fair idea of what is likely to happen in the next birth. It also means that you will have time to change consultants if you feel unhappy about your consultant's position on the management of future deliveries following a caesarean.

When there is a mismatch between the sort of birth you would like — elective caesarean or trial of labour — and the type of delivery your consultant is recommending, it can be very distressing. One woman, who had a very difficult labour followed by an emergency caesarean, was told after the birth that all future births would have to be by caesarean and had mentally prepared herself for this, found that when she subsequently became pregnant her new consultant strongly recommended a trial of labour. She writes:

I was left with the feeling that the control I thought I had had over how my baby was going to be born was rapidly slipping out of my hands.

This situation, where a woman would like an elective caesarean and is being persuaded to have a trial of labour, appears to be less common than the reverse situation, when a woman wants a trial of labour, but her consultant is unwilling or discouraging.

In certain situations you may find it very difficult to find a consultant in favour of a trial of labour, if, for example, you have had two or more caesareans, if you have a classical (vertical) scar or if you have a small pelvis.

In Britain it has been, and largely still is, typical practice for a woman who has had two or more caesareans, even for non-repeating reasons, to be automatically delivered by elective caesarean in any future births. However, not all obstetricians take this view, and it is certainly not a universal policy, as some caesarean mothers have been led to believe. There are a number of recorded cases of women having vaginal births after two or more caesareans, both in Britain[10] and in the USA, where one woman had two vaginal births after four previous caesareans.[11] In Dublin, another woman birthed three of her children vaginally after five caesareans.[12]

The reason why many obstetricians are unwilling to allow a trial of labour after two or more caesareans is that they believe that this increases the likelihood of scar separation. However, recent medical evidence suggests that this belief may well be unfounded, for a number of research studies have been published attesting to the relative safety of trials of labour after two or more caesareans.[13] One of the most comprehensive reviews of the area concluded that, 'While the number of cases is still small, the available evidence does not suggest that a woman who has had more than one previous caesarean section should be treated any differently from the woman who has had only one caesarean,'[14] It is also important to realise that vaginal delivery rates with trials of labour after two or more caesareans are little different from those after just one caesarean; they are estimated to be around 70 per cent.[15] So, there certainly appears to be some medical grounds for challenging the current practice of carrying out repeat caesareans after two or more previous caesarean births.

If you have a classical scar your consultant will, in all probability, strongly advise you against having a trial of labour. This is because classical scars are more likely to separate than the more common lower segment (bikini) variety — studies estimate that around 1 or 2 per cent of classical scars may separate.[16] In addition, the consequences of a classical scar separating are thought to be more serious than if a lower segment scar should separate.[17] However, trials of labour with classical scars are not unheard of.[18] It is also important to realise that a significant proportion of the classical scar separations occur in the last few weeks of pregnancy — in fact, in one study, more than half of all the classical separations arose before the onset of labour[19] — so opting for an elective caesarean is no guarantee that your scar will not separate. One obstetrician believes that if a classical scar is intact at term, then it should withstand labour, since those with questionable integrity usually separate prior to the onset of labour.[20]

Ultimately, the decision to have a trial of labour or an elective caesarean is one that only you and your partner can make, on the basis of all the available medical information. As obstetrician Mitch Levine, who has assisted at a number of vaginal births after classical caesareans, puts it, 'It is my job to explain the risks and benefits to people, not to decide for them.'[21] Similar considerations and risks are thought to apply if you have a vertical scar in the lower part of your uterus, an incision that is sometimes used to deliver premature babies; if your have an 'inverted T' scar that is occasionally necessary if it is difficult to get the baby out through the more usual transverse lower segment incision; or if you have had a hysterotomy (a caesarean operation carried out to terminate a pregnancy, after termination by the usual methods has failed), although there is very little research on these rarer types of scars.[22]

Another situation in which it may be very difficult to find a consultant who supports your desire for a trial of labour is if your first caesarean was carried out for suspected disproportion (when the baby will not fit through your pelvis) or if your pelvic measurements are on the small side. You may well be told that your chances of giving birth vaginally are very low, and that you should therefore have an elective caesarean. But in many cases this is simply not true. Using data from six separate studies, obstetricians Jennifer Davies and John Spencer found that around two-thirds of women whose first caesarean was carried out for disproportion or failure to progress — these two indications are combined because failure to progress is often the way that disproportion presents itself — delivered vaginally following a trial of labour.[23] In the largest study of women with a history of caesarean delivery for disproportion or failure to progress who had a trial of labour, there was an impressive vaginal delivery rate of just over 75 per cent.[24]

You may be told that an x-ray or clinical pelvimetry (estimation of the size of your pelvis by vaginal examination) indicates that the size or shape of your pelvis precludes a vaginal delivery. It is important to realise, however, that such assertions are invariably statements of opinion rather than medical fact. As I discussed in Chapter 1, assuming the baby is not breech, then research clearly indicates that neither x-ray nor clinical pelvimetry can predict disproportion with sufficient accuracy to justify an elective caesarean.[25] Similarly, Jennifer Davies and John Spencer conclude that 'assessment by x-ray pelvimetry does not seem to confer any advantage in the selection of suitable patients for trial of scar'.[26] There are many women, myself included, whose childbirth experiences prove that it is indeed possible to have a vaginal birth after a previous caesarean for suspected disproportion, or with a small pelvis.[27] There are cases of women who have given birth vaginally after being told that they had completely contracted pelvises,[28] and of a woman who birthed a baby weighing over 7 lbs (3 kg), despite her obstetrician's prediction that she would never be able to deliver even a 3 lbs (1.3 kg) baby vaginally.[29]

You may be told that women tend to have larger babies in subsequent pregnancies, that you are unlikely to be able to deliver a larger baby vaginally and that you should therefore opt for an elective caesarean. But not all women have bigger babies second time around. Also, the medical evidence suggests that the fact that a woman is carrying a large baby is not, in itself, a sufficient reason to advise against a trial of labour.[30] It is important to remember that the baby's size is just one factor that can affect whether or not a vaginal birth is possible. Again, there are a number of women who can testify that it is indeed possible to give birth vaginally to babies that are larger than their previous babies delivered by caesarean because of disproportion.[31]

You might also be told that to go into labour when you have

a small pelvis will put undue pressure on your scar, making it more likely to separate. However, this claim is not supported by the available medical evidence. Professor of Obstetrics, Murray Enkin, who has carried out a comprehensive review of research on labour and delivery after a previous caesarean, cites four studies that confirm the safety of trials of labour when the first caesarean was performed for disproportion, and concludes that a history of disproportion or failure to progress is not a contraindication to a trial of labour.[32]

Although most medical evidence suggests that a trial of labour is a sensible course of action, even in cases of suspected disproportion, this remains a contested and controversial issue. Two of the five cases that were put forward as evidence against British obstetrician Wendy Savage, who was suspended from medical practice in 1985, concerned women with suspected disproportion. It was felt that it was inappropriate or dangerous to allow these women to have a trial of labour, but as Wendy Savage points out, it is extremely important to some women to know, with the evidence of their own bodies, that they are not going to deliver vaginally.[33] After a long public enquiry, Wendy Savage's care and practice was vindicated, and her principle stands — that 'a woman should be allowed to have a trial of labour, even if I do not think that she will succeed, as long as she and the baby are all right'.[34]

If you have a small pelvis, if your first caesarean was carried out for suspected disproportion or if the baby you are carrying is large and you wish to have a trial of labour, there are certainly some consultants who would support you in this. Obstetrician Kenneth McKinney, who has assisted at many vaginal births that followed caesareans for disproportion, believes that unless there is an indication in the current pregnancy that a vaginal birth would not be possible, such as placenta praevia, then the woman is a candidate to deliver vaginally. He writes, 'a case could almost be made for making a trial of labour following a previous cesarean mandatory. It probably represents the best obstetrical care for mother and baby.'[35]

There are a number of other situations where consultants are often very discouraging about trials of labour after a previous caesarean. You may find it difficult to obtain a trial of labour if you have had a caesarean and your present baby is breech. This is because the whole subject of breech birth is a contentious one, as discussed in Chapter 1. In addition, some obstetricians are concerned that forceps that are sometimes used to manipulate or 'extract' a breech baby during a vaginal delivery might increase the chances of scar separation.[36] However, there is some debate about whether this is actually the case, for there is, as yet, insufficient evidence on which to recommend or advise against breech trials of labour,[37] and breech VBACs are certainly not unheard of.[38]

You are also likely to meet some resistance if you would like a trial of labour and you are carrying twins.[39] This is because twins are more commonly delivered by caesarean than single babies (see Chapter 1), and because internal manipulation of the second twin is sometimes necessary, a procedure which is thought by some to put undue stress on the caesarean scar. But again, there is thought to be insufficient medical evidence on which to base a recommendation for either a trial of labour or elective caesarean.[40] Consequently, some consultants are willing to allow a trial of labour in this situation, and there have been cases of VBAC twins and even triplets.[41]

You might also be discouraged from having a trial of labour if your baby is overdue. Babies who arrive late tend to be larger and the bones in their head are slightly less malleable and both of these factors may have a small influence on your chances of delivering vaginally. However, it is only rarely that being overdue will tip the balance in favour of an elective caesarean. And, as Elizabeth Shearer points out, 'many doctors . . . require a woman to go into labour by 40 or 41 weeks. Why? Just because she has had a cesarean before — should she be expected to deliver early?'[42]

Another situation where your consultant may be reluctant to allow you to have a trial of labour is if you suffered from a wound infection after your previous caesarean. Infection is believed by some to weaken the scar and make it more prone to separate, but there is, in fact, very little medical evidence to support this view.[43] Some have even speculated that infection might actually strengthen the caesarean scar.[44]

Finally, there are some obstetricians who are unwilling to allow trials of labour when a woman is in her late thirties or early forties,[45] but there appears to be little medical justification for this practice.

By now it should be apparent that you may well need to be very assertive if you would like a trial of labour but you fall into one of the categories described above. One woman whose first baby was born by caesarean due to failure to progress and who had her next three children vaginally, writes:

> If I'd not been so desperate on each occasion to try to have the baby myself I would probably have been given a caesarean for number two and number three, so possibly wouldn't have got as far as number four. So, I think the most important thing when faced with the possibility of a section is to ask, ask, ask, until you have all the information. Sometimes there will be no choice — but there are times when the doctors are able to take account of individual's feelings providing the baby is OK.

If you find yourself in this situation there are a number of things that you can do. It would help if you acquaint yourself with all the relevant medical evidence. Contact those who may be able to support you in your quest — childbirth organisations, caesarean and VBAC support groups, and your local Community Health Council, for example (see pages 237-8 for addresses). Enlist the help of your partner and sympathetic friends. If you have not seen your consultant, ask to see him or her, because a consultant will sometimes be willing to allow a trial of labour when a less senior doctor has recommended a repeat caesarean. Ask your GP to arrange for you to have a second opinion about whether a trial of labour might be possible in your case. Find out the policies of the consultants at your local hospitals. You can do this by either writing to the consultants directly or by contacting the supervisor of midwives or director of midwifery services at the hospital concerned. If necessary, change consultants or hospitals — your GP can arrange this for you.

If you are unable to find a consultant who supports your desire for a trial of labour, remember that, as a last resort, you can simply refuse to have a caesarean. A doctor can refuse to attend you but if you are in hospital the hospital authorities are under an obligation to find another doctor to take his or her place.[46] Such a situation is, however, very unsatisfactory and one to be avoided if at all possible.

TRIALS AND TRIBULATIONS

You may be wondering exactly what a trial of labour involves. There are no definitive answers to this question since opinions differ about the amount of intervention that is necessary or desirable in a trial of labour after a previous caesarean. Occasionally, there will be little to distinguish a trial of labour from other labours:

> In the end everything was very normal and our second daughter arrived quickly into this world with one push. It was just my husband, the midwife and student midwife. No monitors, just the midwife and her trumpet.

In fact, Murray Enkin and his colleagues, who have carried out one of the most comprehensive reviews of practices in childbirth, write, 'The care of a woman in labour after a previous lower segment [horizontal incision] caesarean section should be little different from that for any woman in labour.'[47] Similarly, Elizabeth Shearer, a member of the American National Institute of Health's Task Force of Caesarean Childbirth, believes that, 'there is no more justification for routine intervention [in VBAC labours] than in any other labor'.[48]

However, in Britain, as in a number of other countries, trials of labour do usually involve quite high levels of medical intervention.[49] Typically, a woman having a trial of labour after a caesarean will be expected to have an intravenous drip in place, and to have an electrode attached to her baby's scalp to provide continuous electronic monitoring. Relatively short and arbitrary time limits are also often placed on the trial.

SCAR SEPARATION IN PERSPECTIVE

The main reason why trials of labour are typically not treated like any other labour is because of the spectre of scar separation.

I have chosen to use the term scar separation rather than uterine rupture, since the former term conveys a more accurate picture of what happens in most instances where this problem arises. If a lower segment caesarean scar — the type of scar that the vast majority of caesarean mothers have — comes apart, it is usually a symptomless and benign slow separation, also known as a dehiscence or a window, that causes no problems to mother or baby and does not require treatment,[50] whereas the word rupture conjures up images of wombs ripping apart and almost exploding, with devastating effects. Where a serious separation does occur in a lower segment scar it is rarely catastrophic — massive haemorrhage does not occur but an emergency caesarean will be necessary — and mother and baby are invariably safe.[51]

Scar separation is, in fact, rare. Excluding benign, symptomless separations, reported rates for lower segment scars range from 0.09 per cent, that is less than one in 1,000, to 0.22 per cent, which is around one in 500.[52] As discussed earlier in this chapter, classical scars are slightly more prone to separate.

There are a number of signs that may indicate that scar separation is imminent or has occurred, although many separations are symptomless. These signs include abdominal pain, bleeding from the vagina, swelling over the scar, fever, a uterus that becomes and remains rigid, shock, a raised pulse rate followed by a drop in blood pressure[53] and changes in the baby's heart rate.[54] However, not all of these symptoms are definitive signs of scar separation. Abdominal pain, for example, is an unreliable indicator, for some separations are painless,[55] and in one study of twenty repeat caesareans performed because of severe lower abdominal pain, only one scar separation was found.[56] If you do experience pain in this area it certainly does not necessarily mean that your scar has separated and that you will need to have an emergency caesarean. You would, however, be well advised to contact the hospital so that your condition and that of your baby can be checked to make sure that all is well.

Although the prospect of scar separation is very worrying to some women, a concern that also often appears to be uppermost in the minds of those caring for women in labour after a previous caesarean, it is important to put the problem of scar separation into some sort of perspective. Perhaps the most important thing to remember is that the risks to both yourself and your baby are greater if you opt for an elective repeat caesarean (assuming that there is no indication for a caesarean in your present pregnancy) than if you decide to have a trial of labour.[57] This is because scar separation makes only a tiny contribution to the overall incidence of perinatal and maternal mortality for women undergoing a trial of labour, and because elective caesarean delivery carries its own, albeit small, risks which more than counterbalance the risks of scar separation.[58] It is also important to realise that a significant minority of lower segment scar separations and over half of all classical scar separations, occur during late pregnancy rather than during labour itself, and so would probably not have been prevented by an elective caesarean.[59] In addition, it is helpful to remember that over half of all cases of uterine rupture involve women who have never had a caesarean delivery.[60]

Considering these facts, it could be argued that the way trials of labour after a caesarean are typically managed is an over-reaction to a minimal risk. It is a question of the balance of risks. Some of the interventions common in trials of labour, described below, are not in themselves risk-free. They can also sometimes have a deleterious effect on labour, thereby necessitating a caesarean which might otherwise have been avoided, so the risks of an avoidable caesarean birth must also be taken into consideration. This is one of the reasons why consultants differ in the level of intervention that they recommend.

DEGREES OF INTERVENTION

Some obstetricians will suggest that you come into hospital at the very beginning of labour, others will be happy for you to stay at home until you feel ready to come in, but perhaps the majority will advise you to come in relatively early in labour. The advantage of going to hospital early is that if a problem with your scar should arise during the early stages of labour you are in the best place for it to be dealt with. A possible disadvantage of going into hospital early in labour is that you may feel less relaxed there and this could affect the progress of your labour. In fact, research indicates that those who go into hospital sooner rather than later are more likely to have a caesarean delivery.[61] You may, depending on provision and policy in your local area, be able to have a domino delivery — a number of women with previous caesareans have done so. In a domino delivery, one of the midwives who provided your antenatal care visits you at home during early labour, stays with you until it is time to go into hospital, comes with you into hospital and continues looking after you there. If all goes well and you do not need a caesarean she brings you and the baby home a few hours after the birth.

Many obstetricians believe that women having a trial of labour after a previous caesarean should have continuous electronic monitoring. In an informal survey by the Caesarean Support Network, the majority of consultants insisted on this.[62] Many favoured continuous internal monitoring which involves artificially rupturing your membranes (breaking the waters) and clipping an electrode onto your baby's scalp. Some consultants were willing to allow the continuous monitoring to be external, by a monitor attached to a belt strapped around your abdomen, and a handful indicated that monitoring would only be intermittent.

There are two reasons why obstetricians tend to advocate continuous electronic monitoring. Firstly, it may give more information about the baby's condition than intermittent external monitoring by sonicaid (a hand-held monitor that records the baby's heart rate) or fetal stethoscope. Secondly, it may pick up changes in the baby's heart rate that are sometimes an indication of problems in the scar.

However, it is unclear how such changes might be differentiated from changes that reflect mild or transient fetal distress. It is also important to remember that the routine use of continuous electronic monitoring has a number of disadvantages. As discussed in Chapter 1, this type of monitoring tends to immobilise women which can prolong labour and may precipitate fetal distress; the artificial rupture of membranes that is necessary when internal monitoring is used is thought to increase the likelihood of the baby becoming distressed; fetal heart tracings are notoriously difficult to interpret; the medical evidence suggests that intermittent monitoring is equally effective at preventing neonatal death or handicap; and the use of continuous electronic monitoring significantly increases caesarean section rates. You may be interested to know that, having considered all the available evidence, the panel of the Canadian Consensus Conference on Aspects of Caesarean Birth concluded that, 'Continuous electronic monitoring of the fetal heart rate is not routinely indicated [in trials of labour after a previous caesarean].'[63] They do, however, point out that regular checks of the baby's heart rate, by sonicaid or fetal stethoscope, are essential in trials of labour, as they are in any other labour.

Occasionally, women having trials of labour after a previous caesarean are monitored very intensively by means of a device known as an intrauterine catheter which is inserted into the uterus to measure the strength of contractions. This practice is not widespread, but some consultants feel that it provides useful extra information, particularly when labour is induced or accelerated.

Once in hospital, you might also be advised to have an intravenous drip (IV) inserted into your hand — around half of the consultants in the Caesarean Support Network's survey required this.[64] There are two possible reasons why women undergoing trials of labour after a caesarean might be advised to have an IV. The main reason is that in the unlikely event that you scar should separate, there is an even smaller possibility that you might bleed profusely, go into shock and your veins shrivel up. If this should happen it would be difficult to insert a drip, so it is thought to be useful to have a drip already in place. However, it is extremely rare for women to go into shock if a lower segment scar separates. It is true that if an unscarred uterus ruptures there is massive haemorrhage and rapidly advancing shock, but the situation where a previous lower segment caesarean scar separates is very different — bleeding tends to be minimal and mother and baby are invariably fine.[65] Also, as Nancy Cohen and Lois Estner point out, there is a procedure known as 'cut down' that can be used to remedy the situation in the unlikely event that a vein does shrivel.[66]

One other purported reason for having an IV during a trial of labour is to provide nourishment and fluids during the trial since you are unlikely to be allowed to eat or drink once you are in hospital, a policy which is discussed below. However, since it is rare for any woman in labour, whether or not she has previously had a caesarean, to be permitted to eat while in hospital, and since there will typically be quite short time limits on your trial of labour, there does not appear to be any justification for singling out women with previous caesareans for routine intravenous nourishment.

Some women feel reassured by the presence of an IV, but there are some disadvantages. It tends to restrict mobility, and you may be unable to put pressure on the hand in which the drip is inserted which can limit the positions you adopt during labour. You may be offered the compromise of having a cannula (also known as a venflon catheter) put in your hand to keep a vein ready. This solves the mobility problem but not the problem of being unable to put pressure on the hand.

The majority of obstetricians hold the view that a woman who has previously had a caesarean should not be allowed to eat during labour, although women may be permitted to suck ice cubes or to have sips of water.[67] The reason for this policy is that if a caesarean under general anaesthetic becomes necessary then there is a danger that you might vomit and inhale the gastric contents, a problem that is referred to as aspiration or Mendelson's syndrome. This problem is very rare, but is serious, and has been a cause of maternal deaths.

However, it is unclear as to whether restricting labouring women's food intake is the best way to minimise the risks of aspiration. It has long been known that the main cause of maternal deaths from aspiration is the failure to apply proper anaesthetic technique.[68] It is also important to note that withholding food and drink during labour does not guarantee that the stomach will be empty should a general anaesthetic become necessary, that the gastric juices of an empty stomach can be very damaging if inhaled and that deaths from aspiration do not appear to have decreased since the policy of fasting women in labour has been instituted.[69] In addition, fasting can present its own risks to mother and baby — it can lead to dehydration and ketosis (a situation where lactic acid accumulates in the mother's body tissues and fluids, altering the chemistry of her blood and weakening her muscle cells). Ketosis can be detected by checking the mother's urine, and corrected by giving glucose and water intravenously, but this can sometimes have serious, unwanted effects on the baby.[70]

Therefore it is, once again, a question of the balance of risks. In view of the medical evidence, a few hospitals now allow women classified as being at 'low risk' of needing general anaesthesia to eat a light, low-fat diet such as tea, fruit juice, toast, honey and plain biscuits.[71] With a history of caesarean delivery, you are unlikely to be seen as being at low risk of needing another caesarean. But, then again, some might argue that the VBAC rate of around 80 per cent is not so dissimilar to the vaginal delivery rate for women who have not previously given birth by caesarean.

Occasionally, a woman having a trial of labour after a caesarean will have the top part of her pubic hair shaved off, in readiness, should another caesarean become necessary. There appears to be little justification for this practice, since it is highly unlikely that such a dire emergency will arise that the minute or so it takes to carry out the partial shave becomes crucial. In addition, research suggests that it is best to delay shaving until immediately before a caesarean to minimise the risk of infection.[72]

One other aspect that differentiates trials of labour from other labours is the fact that they are usually subject to quite short and arbitrary time limits. The women in my research who had trials of labour after a caesarean were allowed trials of labour varying in length from four hours to twenty-four hours. More typical time limits, however, are eight or twelve hours. A few obstetricians do not set time limits, but, at present, they are in the minority. One reason why time limits are set is because it is felt that a long labour will put an excessive strain on the caesarean scar, making it more likely to separate. It is unclear, however, whether this is medical fact or speculation, since there appears to be very little research on this matter. It would, of course, be difficult to carry out such research nowadays when so few women are allowed to labour for more than twelve hours after a previous caesarean. The one piece of research that I did locate concluded that scar separation was not more likely after a long trial of labour.[73] Time constraints on trials of labour may also reflect the growing tendency for time limits to be placed on all labours, regardless of whether the woman has previously had a caesarean delivery. See Chapter 1 for discussion of the advantages and disadvantages of such policies.

The time limits discussed so far are those given for the first (dilation of the cervix) stage and the second (pushing) stage combined. Most obstetricians also place limits on the length of the second stage in trials of labour after a caesarean (many also place time limits on the second stage for all women in labour). Such limits can vary by anything from thirty minutes to two hours. This is because some obstetricians believe that prolonged pushing can put undue stress on the scar, but again, little research has been carried out on this. In fact, in at least one piece of research all the scar separations occurred during the first stage of labour. [74]

It can be very distressing for a woman to have a repeat caesarean simply because she ran out of time. Time limits can be particularly problematic if your first caesarean was an elective one carried out before the onset of labour. Although it is your second experience of childbirth, as far as labour is concerned, you are a first-time mother and first labours tend to be slower than later ones. Time pressure itself may prolong labour since psychological stress can have powerful physical effects on the body. In their VBAC antenatal classes, Nancy Cohen and Lois Estner illustrate this point dramatically by taking out a stopwatch and a knife, and challenging the males in the room to get an erection and ejaculate within two minutes, or else have the tips of their penises cut off! [75] We can all imagine the effect that such threats would have on a man's ability to have an erection. Some women may find that the pressure to dilate within set time constraints, and the threat of another caesarean if they do not, has a similar effect on their labour.

If you give birth vaginally after a previous caesarean, your doctor may wish to insert his or her hand into your uterus to check the condition of your scar. Some, but by no means all, obstetricians advocate routine manual exploration of the uterus after VBAC deliveries, however all the medical evidence suggests that this practice is unwarranted. [76] It confers no benefit since, in the absence of other signs of scar separation, any small holes or dehiscences that are found will not need treating. Manual exploration of the uterus also carries the risk of introducing infection or of converting a dehiscence into a serious separation.

I should also mention that there are two forms of intervention that are sometimes used less frequently or more cautiously in trials of labour after a caesarean than in other labours. In the past, many obstetricians were reluctant to allow women in labour after a caesarean to have an epidural, because they feared that it might mask the pain or tenderness that sometimes occur before a scar separates. However, the medical research indicates that the pain of a serious separation tends to be felt even through an epidural, and that withholding epidural analgesia in trials of labour is not justified.[77] Nowadays, the majority of consultants appear to be happy to allow women having a trial of labour after a caesarean to have an epidural. There has also been some debate over the use of oxytocin (a drug given intravenously to stimulate or strengthen contractions) to induce or accelerate labour in women who have had a previous caesarean. Some obstetricians believe that its use increases the risk of scar separation, but research indicates that any increased risk is likely to be small.[78] Consequently, many obstetricians now give oxytocin in trials of labour where they feel that induction is necessary or that labour needs to be speeded up.

Many women do not realise all that a trial of labour typically involves until they are well into their next pregnancy, and sometimes not until they are actually in labour. As caesarean mother and campaigner for low intervention trials of labour Yvonne Williams asks, 'after a caesarean section, how many women are told before they leave hospital that their next labour will be a trial?'.[79] High levels of intervention can leave women feeling that they themselves are on trial:

> I strongly resent the implication that the integrity or physiology of my body is faulty. I can accept intervention as a solution to a problem, but not the undermining attitude that I must 'perform' to a specified level within a set time scale as though I had to prove something or pass an exam.

Consultants do differ in the amount and types of intervention they require and there are some who advocate minimum intervention trials of labour, so it is well worth finding out your consultant's policy and questioning interventions that you feel are unwarranted. Some women are happy to have high intervention trials of labour, others are not — ultimately it must be your decision.

If you would like a low-intervention trial of labour, but are having difficulty in obtaining one, it can be very frustrating. There are, however, a number of things that you can do. The suggestions made earlier in this chapter regarding obtaining a trial of labour also apply to those endeavouring to obtain a low-intervention trial of labour — do not battle on alone: find some support; ask to see your consultant; question him or her — there is sometimes room for negotiation; be assertive; find out the policies of other consultants in your area; ask for a second opinion; and remember that, if all else fails, you have the right to refuse medical intervention.[80] It is, nevertheless, sad that caesarean mothers sometimes have to go through this battle to get a low-intervention trial of labour:

> While I appreciate the consultant's clear explanation of the procedure for a trial of labour, I am now bracing myself either to submit to the rigid protocol of managed labour and birth within time constraints, or argue the process with the consultant — something I could do without. I feel my energies and emotions should be directed more positively than defending my rights and wishes to have a minimum intervention labour.

HOME BIRTH

So far I have discussed birth after a caesarean in terms of elective caesareans and high- and low-intervention trials of labour, but there is a fourth option, albeit one taken by only a tiny minority of caesarean mothers, and that is home birth. Most obstetricians would advise you against this option, in the strongest possible terms, mainly because of the risk of scar separation. Although any woman has the right to have her baby at home, whatever her obstetric history, you are likely to meet with considerable opposition if you request a home birth after a previous caesarean. A number of women have, nevertheless, given birth at home after a previous caesarean delivery.[81]

It is not a decision to be taken lightly, as one woman who had a VBAC at home writes:

After reading all the available literature and very careful consideration, we decided the risks involved did not outweigh the benefits of a home birth ... We made it clear that the responsibility was ours and that we had made an informed decision. [82]

Childbirth writer Nicky Wesson, who has herself had a home birth after a previous caesarean, lists a number of possible reasons for having a baby at home after encountering difficulties with a previous birth. She believes that you are likely to feel relaxed in your own surroundings; you will be more able to adopt any position that you instinctively feel will help the baby out; it is unlikely that there will be an atmosphere of controlled impatience and eagerness to get it all over and done with; you will have continuity of care; and there will be less routine medical intervention. [83]

If you are considering having a home birth you may find it helpful to contact the Society to Support Home Confinement (see page 238 for address). Nicky Wesson suggests that you consider contacting an independent midwife if you would like a home birth and are considered 'high risk', as caesarean mothers typically are. [84] Independent midwives are independent practitioners who care for women antenatally, during labour and delivery and postnatally (whose services you have to pay for), and are sometimes more willing and confident than community midwives about booking a woman for a home delivery after a previous caesarean (see page 238 for address). Independent midwives are also sometimes able to provide care during labour and delivery if you wish to have your baby in hospital.

CAESAREAN BIRTH SECOND TIME AROUND

Caesarean birth can be a much more positive experience second (or third or fourth) time around. In my research, women were less likely to suffer from postnatal depression after a subsequent caesarean than after a first caesarean. They were also less likely to have difficulties in forming a relationship with their baby after a subsequent caesarean.[85] Interestingly, there were no differences between those who had had just one caesarean and those who had had more than one in the extent to which they had difficult feelings about the birth, a finding that is echoed in other research.[86] Nevertheless, some women do find second caesareans much more satisfying and less distressing than first caesareans. This is particularly so when the first caesarean was carried out under general anaesthetic and the second one with regional anaesthesia:

> My first caesarean was with a general anaesthetic and the second was with an epidural. The contrast could not have been greater. Physically and emotionally after the general anaesthetic I was a wreck. After the epidural I was on cloud nine!

> It was indescribably euphoric to actually 'be there' at the birth.

> For some reason, having been there awake for his delivery made me feel better about the whole experience of caesarean birth. It is as if at last I've almost got it right!

Having had a caesarean once before, the experience is one that you know something about, and you are less likely to be left with the sense of shock that is common after first-time emergency caesareans.

> A second caesarean is easier as you know what to expect and the fear is less.

Knowing that another caesarean is a possibility or that you will definitely give birth by caesarean this time enables you to prepare yourself, something you may have been unable to do first time around. This preparation can make all the difference. One woman described how she prepared herself for her second caesarean as follows:

> I knew at 18 weeks that I was going to have a planned elective caesarean under epidural, which I had chosen so that my

husband could be with me all the way. I tried to make sure I was well prepared and had a positive attitude. To do this I began yoga classes which I found a great help in calming my mind and body in the long wait before and during the operation itself. I also got a book on caesareans from the library and hired a video of a caesarean birth under epidural from the National Caesarean Support Network, who were very helpful. I also had some Bach Flower Remedies made up especially for me and my feelings towards the situation. I also took some homoeopathic remedies for nerves, pain and for healing wounds which I found beneficial . . . I now feel that this second birth experience has been so much happier for me and my husband than the first caesarean, and feel that this is mostly due to the fact that I was prepared mentally and physically.

Something else that can help to make a subsequent caesarean a more positive experience is the fact that, having already experienced caesarean birth, you will have a better idea of what you would find helpful and will be more able to ask for what you need:

Overall the pregnancy and birth was fine, it was the postnatal care that was lacking and unsatisfactory. I have identified ways to do things differently postnatally if I have to have another caesarean — I will pay for a single amenity room if one is available (much against my socialist principles) or will ask for an early discharge once I'm off painkilling injections.

A variety of caesarean birth options are listed in Chapter 10 — things that some women have found helpful and that you may wish to consider requesting in your next caesarean birth.

Several women commented that their physical recovery was easier and quicker second time around, although a few found it more difficult to find the time to rest, having a toddler to care for as well as a new baby.

You may wonder what your scar will look like after two or more caesareans. Some women find that their scar is more noticeable or less neat after two or more caesareans, but others feel that its appearance improves and comment that it was 'tidied up' second time around. Scars themselves vary, as does the way different women perceive their scars, but caesarean mothers do not appear to be any more likely to dislike their scars after two or more caesareans than they are after just one.[87]

The way women feel after a subsequent caesarean will vary depending not only on the type of anaesthesia used, but also on whether the caesarean was elective or was carried out after a trial of labour. Some women feel very happy about delivering by caesarean after a 'failed' trial of labour, particularly when the labour was a positive experience and the caesarean was perceived to have been necessary and unavoidable. Sometimes, however, women can feel very disappointed:

> I was asked at 38 weeks of pregnancy what I would like to do. I opted for a trial of labour. I was so pleased, I thought I could prove myself and do it all 'properly'. It was not to be. My second son got stuck when I was almost 10 cm dilated. I was even more disappointed this time — so close but so far.

This sense of disappointment can be profound. One caesarean mother whose second child was born by caesarean after a trial of labour, wrote:

> I woke up from the anaesthetic and the next thing I knew I was hearing myself crying. I didn't know why I was crying, but then as the days passed I realised that maybe it was my soul crying. When I went home on the fifth day all I could think about was having another baby, really having one, myself . . . My third child was born by caesarean after another trial of labour. When I came home I seemed all right, I suppose, not so many tears as before, but inside was a feeling of great loss and sadness, it was like a silent ache that was just with me everywhere. I'm not at present thinking of having any more children, but somewhere at the back of my mind is the thought that maybe, some day, I might again try for my greatest wish, to give birth.

Feelings — of disappointment, failure and anger — are more likely to surface when a woman feels that her caesarean was unnecessary or avoidable, that she has not been given a fair trial:

> It was like the staff were waiting eagerly for a tiny sign to carry out another caesarean. When I was admitted the midwife had part shaved me as a precaution for being ready for another caesarean. I felt like I was being patronised and that the staff were all saying what they felt I wanted to hear, but were in fact going to do what they wanted to do all along.

Like perceptions of necessity, a feeling of being involved in decisions and a sense of autonomy is another crucial element in determining the way women feel about subsequent caesareans. One caesarean mother who, in the event, gave birth vaginally second time around, writes:

> I had to rid myself of the feeling that another caesarean would be a 'failure'. The important thing would be that next time I would be in control and making the best choice I could. The actual method of delivery would not be the be-all and end-all. I think the crucial factor is to do with power and control. I prepared myself mentally for the possibility that I might need another caesarean, but it would be because I needed one, not because it was forced on me.

The amount and type of care and support given during a trial of labour and caesarean birth can also have a major influence on the way women feel about their experience:

> My first caesarean was altogether an unsatisfactory experience. My second caesarean was completely different, despite another twenty-four hour labour and the baby turning to posterior again. They were on my side, the whole thing was managed well, with my input being accepted, and finally the decision to deliver under epidural — well, it was a triumph. I felt we had all done our best, but that the caesar was necessary. Being wide awake and involved throughout, this positive experience finally laid to rest all the frustrations and anger of the first go.

THE VBAC EXPERIENCE

Like the positive experience of a second caesarean birth above, a vaginal birth after a caesarean has enormous potential for 'laying to rest' the painful feelings arising from a difficult caesarean experience. For many women, a vaginal birth is the final step in the long process of coming to terms with their caesarean — the experience that finally heals the wound in the mind. VBAC mothers describe feeling 'whole', 'normal', 'female once more', 'strengthened' and 'healed'.[88]

Not all VBACs are wonderful. Those factors — perceptions of necessity, involvement and support — that shape the way a woman feels about her caesarean experience, also play a role in vaginal birth. If a woman in labour is subjected to interventions that she feels are unnecessary, if procedures are carried out without her consent, if she is given little information about what is happening, if decisions are made over her head, if she feels disempowered and debased, and if she is not treated with care, sensitivity and respect, then her experience of childbirth, whether vaginal or caesarean, will not be a positive one. And, even when the VBAC experience is positive, as Nancy Cohen and Lois Estner point out, the joy of the VBAC can sometimes make the pain of the caesarean more difficult to bear.[89]

Nevertheless, I would like to end this chapter with the words of VBAC mothers who describe the joy, sense of accomplishment and euphoria that a vaginal birth after a caesarean can bring:

A forceps delivery under epidural is not the best delivery, but it felt like heaven.

Elizabeth arrived very speedily after a three-hour, relatively painless labour. Her delivery made up for all the disappointment and anguish I suffered after Helen's birth.

It was over — the baby was born — I can't describe the tremendous feelings of relief, happiness, fulfilment. I couldn't believe I'd done it myself. It was amazing to be able to get up and walk almost straight away and to get a shower. The physical recovery was totally different. This really does help a lot.

It was worth all the pain — to get it over with before the birth rather than having it afterwards. I was so pleased with myself for having managed it the 'right' way this time that I couldn't sleep all night.

My son's birth turned out better than my wildest dreams, as I had a quick, easy labour with a wonderful midwife who wasn't the least bit rattled by the scar in my uterus. I had no IV drip, no continuous monitoring or pain relief and a natural third stage. The emotional and psychological sequelae of my second birth were astoundingly different from my first. After the caesarean, I suffered from postnatal depression, this time I 'suffered' from postnatal euphoria which is only just wearing off. I'm glad I plucked up the courage to have a second baby, as this second experience has healed so many wounds and laid so many 'ghosts' to rest.

10 What is to be Done

In this final chapter we turn to the question of what we, as expectant mothers and consumers of maternity care, can do, both to minimise our chances of needing a caesarean, and when a caesarean is necessary, to help to make the experience a positive and happy one. I then bring the book to a close by outlining what health professionals can do to meet the needs of caesarean mothers and to help to ensure that every caesarean is a good caesarean.

CAESAREAN PREVENTION

It is with some trepidation that I broach the subject of caesarean prevention. I am very aware that to suggest that some caesareans may be avoided or prevented may only serve to increase the feelings of self-blame, of 'if only I'd done this', 'if only I hadn't done that' which many women experience after a caesarean birth. If reading this section makes you feel that way, then I can only say that this was not my intention and that I am sorry. What we must remember is that all mothers do their very best, given their own physical and emotional resources, and the support available to them, and every mother makes decisions based on what she believes to be in the best interests of her baby and herself. Those looking after us also invariably acted out of their genuine concern for us and our babies. Although, with hindsight, we might wish that we had done things differently, we cannot change the past. It is time to forgive ourselves and those who provided our maternity care.

It is also important to realise that there is no way of knowing whether a different course of action would have resulted in a different outcome — a caesarean might still have been needed. A small number of caesareans will always be necessary. Even Michel Odent's maternity unit in Pithiviers, France, which has been held up as a model of good practice and low-intervention childbirth, has a caesarean birth rate of 5 per cent.[1]

Caesarean prevention can begin in pregnancy. Although there is actually very little medical evidence linking nutrition and exercise during pregnancy with type of delivery or conditions necessitating a caesarean, common sense suggests that it is a good idea to eat a healthy, balanced diet and to keep relatively fit during pregnancy. If you are planning to have an active birth (that is one in which you follow your own instincts, are mobile and adopt upright positions such as standing, kneeling or squatting), it is advisable to practice some yoga-based exercises, such as squatting, during your pregnancy in preparation for the birth.[2]

It is important to take care in choosing the best and most appropriate place for you to give birth. Consider the alternatives: a hospital delivery (which hospital? which consultant?); a domino delivery where the same community midwife looks after you during labour at home, brings you to hospital for the birth and takes you and your baby home soon afterwards; birth in a GP unit (a hospital or ward where care is provided by an obstetric GP and community midwives); or a home birth. Research suggests that caesarean delivery rates tend to be lower when women of equivalent risk status are cared for by midwives or GPs,[3] and obstetricians have even been cited as a 'risk factor for caesarean delivery'.[4]

Generalisations are unwise, however, and the best place for you to give birth will depend on the type and quality of care on offer, your own particular preferences and your individual medical circumstances and obstetric history. You may wish to find out which hospital, or consultant, in your area has a low caesarean delivery rate. You may have some difficulty ascertaining this, since hospitals are not obliged to produce such statistics and many are unwilling to release them if they have them. If the hospital is not forthcoming, you could try asking your local Community Health Council if they have such information. Remember that maternity statistics need to be interpreted with some caution since rates will vary according to the population a unit serves and the number of high-risk women referred or transferred to a particular unit;

therefore a high caesarean rate does not necessarily mean that too many caesareans are being carried out. Childbirth organisations and local childbirth teachers may also be able to give you some information about the policies and general orientation of various hospitals and consultants in your locality.

If you are told during pregnancy that an elective caesarean is necessary, ask exactly why this is so in your case. If the reason for the proposed elective caesarean falls into one of the 'grey areas' where obstetric opinion differs about the best course of action, such as breech births, suspected disproportion and repeat caesareans (see Chapters 1 and 9), ask if a trial of labour might be possible. Also, remember that you are entitled to a second opinion — ask your GP to arrange this for you, if you would like one.

If your baby is breech, ask whether external version — where the obstetrician turns the baby by gently manipulating your abdomen — might be possible. There are also various exercises that you might like to try to encourage your baby to turn to a head-down position. Janet Balaskas suggests lying on your back with a number of pillows under your bottom, so that your pelvis is higher than your head, and relaxing in this position for ten minutes several times a day. [5] She recommends that you discuss it with your midwife or doctor before embarking on this exercise and that you stop if it makes you feel dizzy. An alternative breech-turning exercise is described by Sheila Kitzinger — this involves kneeling, with your chest and abdomen resting on a beanbag on the floor and your bottom in the air, higher than your head, for twenty to thirty minutes several times a day. [6] Walking for an hour a day is also thought to encourage a breech baby to turn. [7]

If your baby is in a posterior position, with his back lying against yours and his limbs facing your abdominal wall, this can prolong labour and a caesarean delivery is sometimes needed. You can encourage a posterior baby to change to the more usual anterior position by adopting leaning forward positions or kneeling on all fours during late pregnancy and labour. [8]

If you are told that your baby needs to be induced it is important to ask whether this is absolutely necessary in your case. Research suggests that there is no justification for inducing babies simply because they are a few days late, and there is, at present, not enough evidence to indicate whether induction or a wait-and-see policy is best when a baby is more than two weeks overdue.[9] Induction is not always successful and failed induction was the fifth most common reason for caesareans amongst the women in my research. Although there is little evidence of a direct association between induction and caesarean delivery rates,[10] it is probably best to avoid being induced unless it is absolutely necessary since, as discussed in Chapter 1, induction can be the first step in a cascade of intervention that leads to prolonged labour or fetal distress, thereby necessitating a caesarean.

When you are in labour it is important to think carefully about when is the best time to go into hospital. Research suggests that women who go into hospital early on in labour are more likely to have a caesarean than those who go to hospital at a later stage in labour.[11] It is also important that you have good care and support during labour. Some studies have found that the presence of a supportive companion during labour results in fewer caesarean deliveries.[12] Sometimes your partner, along with your midwife, will be able to provide all the care and support you need, but some women find it helpful to have a female friend or 'birth attendant' with them during labour in addition to their partner and professional carers.[13]

It would certainly be a good idea to keep mobile during labour, to walk around and change position frequently. Upright positions — standing, kneeling, leaning forward, sitting upright or squatting — are recommended. Avoid lying on your back as this tends to prolong labour and may precipitate fetal distress.[14] If you need to lie down to rest or sleep it is best to lie on your side. Research suggests that being mobile and upright increases the intensity and efficiency of contractions, is less painful, decreases the need for analgesics, makes both the first and second stages of labour shorter and tends to make fetal distress less likely.[15] Since fetal distress and prolonged labour are common reasons for carrying out a caesarean, it makes sense to remain mobile and upright. Disproportion is another common reason for having a caesarean birth. By squatting you can increase the diameters of your pelvis by as much as 30 per cent,[16] maximising the chances that your baby will be able to fit through your pelvis, and minimising your chances of needing a caesarean for disproportion.

It would also be wise to avoid routine intervention in labour, such as the artificial rupture of membranes (breaking the bag of waters that surrounds the baby), acceleration of labour by use of intravenous oxytocin and continuous electronic monitoring. Whilst there are certainly some situations in which these interventions are necessary and invaluable, to use them as a matter of course in a normal labour does not appear to be warranted and may increase your chances of needing a caesarean.

Research indicates that whilst artificially rupturing the membranes may well speed up labour, will reveal whether meconium is present in the waters, which can be a sign that the baby is distressed, and is necessary (unless the membranes have already ruptured spontaneously) if continuous internal monitoring is to be used, there is as yet little evidence that the procedure confers more benefit than harm.[17] Indeed, some research suggests that artificially rupturing the membranes can have adverse effects on the baby's heart rate, although no large randomised trials have yet been carried out to confirm or refute this.[18]

Similarly, whilst the use of oxytocin to speed up a labour that is progressing slowly can be very helpful in some cases, and result in a vaginal birth when a caesarean might otherwise have been needed, its routine or liberal use may cause more problems than it solves. Some research suggests an association between the use of oxytocin and fetal distress.[19] Moreover, Murray Enkin and his colleagues conclude that the liberal use of oxytocin does not appear to be of benefit to mothers or babies, and point out that encouraging women to get up and move around, stand or sit as they wish, can be more effective in speeding up labour than giving oxytocin.[20]

You might also want to avoid the routine use of continuous electronic monitoring. Although it is vital that your baby's heart rate is monitored during labour, in the majority of cases this can be done just as effectively by regular checks using a fetal stethoscope or hand-held ultrasound monitor (sonicaid).[21] Of course, there are some situations where continuous electronic monitoring may well be advisable, such as if oxytocin is used to stimulate or accelerate your labour, if it is a multiple pregnancy or if there is meconium-staining in the fluid that surrounds the baby, but if your labour does not fall into one of these categories continuous monitoring does not appear to be warranted.[22] As discussed in Chapter 1, the routine use of continuous electronic monitoring has been found to significantly increase caesarean birth rates.[23] This may be because it tends to immobilise women and restrict the positions that they may adopt, and this may precipitate fetal distress or prolong labour and result in a caesarean delivery. It may also be because the tracings of this type of monitoring are very difficult to interpret, and both their ambiguity and permanence may encourage defensive medicine and early resort to caesarean delivery. If your baby is showing signs of fetal distress, try changing to a different position as babies' heart rates have been known to return to normal simply as a result of a change in maternal position. In addition, if your baby's heart rate is giving cause for concern, it is well worth asking whether a fetal scalp blood sample could be taken to verify the diagnosis of fetal distress and confirm the necessity for a caesarean delivery.

It is also important to think carefully about what type of pain relief to have during labour. Types of pain relief that are not thought to increase the chances of a caesarean becoming necessary include entonox (a mixture of gas and oxygen that is breathed in through a mask just before and during contractions) and TENS (transcutaneous electrical nerve stimulation). A TENS machine consists of a small hand-held box which generates low-voltage electrical impulses which are sent along wires to pads attached to the mother's back, and the mother herself can alter the frequency and intensity of the impulses as labour progresses. Other things that some women have found helpful in relieving pain during labour include walking around, taking a bath, listening to music, breathing techniques, massage and hypnosis, none of which are likely to increase your chances of needing a caesarean. Whilst pain-relieving medication such as pethidine and epidural analgesia can be of great benefit, they also have some drawbacks. Some research suggests that pethidine can slow down labour, although the evidence for this is not conclusive.[24] You may also want to avoid epidural analgesia since it appears, in some instances, to be implicated in fetal distress.[25] Furthermore, although there is little direct evidence to link epidurals and caesareans, Doris Haire, the President of the American Foundation for Maternal and Child Health, asserts, 'Most obstetricians quietly agree that epidural block also increases the rate of cesarean section.'[26] However, the possible disadvantages of epidurals have to be set against the potential benefits. Over and above its pain-relieving properties, there is the advantage that by having an epidural set up during labour, you increase your chances of being able to have epidural anaesthesia, rather than a general anaesthetic, should a caesarean later prove necessary.

Given the present state of obstetric knowledge and the fact that caesarean prevention is a relatively new and uncharted field, a number of the suggestions that I have given for minimising your chances of needing a caesarean are somewhat speculative and may need revising in the light of future research. They are, however, useful starting points in the quest to make every caesarean a necessary and unavoidable caesarean.

HELPING YOURSELF TO A BETTER CAESAREAN

Preparation and information can make an enormous difference to the way a caesarean birth is experienced. Read everything that you can find on it. If caesareans are not covered in your antenatal classes, bring up the topic yourself. Talk to other caesarean parents you know. Make contact with your local caesarean support group. They will be able to share their experiences of caesarean birth with you, but remember that your own experience may well be very different. You will also be able to talk through any worries you may have. Most groups have a library of books, leaflets and articles to provide further information. Some groups also show or lend out videos of caesarean births. Ask questions about caesareans at your antenatal appointments — you may find it helpful to take along a list of your questions. Do not feel that you are unnecessarily taking up the midwife's or doctor's time — providing information about what will happen to you is as much part of your medical care as checking your weight and blood pressure. As one caesarean mother put it:

Mums should ask, ask, ask about anything and everything whilst pregnant and during the birth.

It is also a good idea to consider carefully all the alternatives that are open to you. Not all caesarean births are carried out in the same way, and caesarean mothers differ in their needs and preferences. Below is a list of options for caesarean birth that you might like to think about. The list is not exhaustive or immutable — its purpose is merely to encourage you to think about what you, your partner and your soon-to-be-born baby need to help make your caesarean experience a positive and happy one. Unfortunately, there is no guarantee that all these options will be available at the hospital where you are to have your baby. Sometimes, there will be medical reasons why a particular option is not open to you; and sometimes options will not be on offer for financial or practical reasons or because of a consultant's personal preferences or hospital policy. If your request for a particular alternative is declined due to hospital policy or the consultant's preferences, you may well have a case to argue. If the answer is still no, it is well worth considering changing to another consultant or to another hospital where your needs and preferences can be accommodated.

There are a number of steps you can take to find out the policies of other consultants or hospitals in your area. Your GP may be able to discover this information for you. You could try writing to the consultants yourself, or you could contact the supervisor of midwives, or director of midwifery services, at the hospital concerned. Childbirth organisations, caesarean support groups or your local Community Health Council may also be able to provide you with information on alternatives available at different hospitals, and support in your search for a hospital that can meet your needs. Even if you are unsuccessful, the very fact that you asked will have helped to generate a greater awareness of the many and diverse needs of caesarean parents. And by making our wishes known we may play a part in changing practices, so that one day all the alternatives listed here will be offered as a matter of course.

CAESAREAN BIRTH ALTERNATIVES

- If there is some doubt about whether or not a caesarean will be necessary, you could opt for an elective caesarean or a trial of labour.
- If you are to have an elective caesarean, this could be carried out on a date agreed upon in advance or you could wait until labour begins.
- If your caesarean is scheduled for a particular date, you could be admitted to hospital the night before or you could go in on the morning of the operation.
- The caesarean could be carried out with a general anaesthetic, or with epidural or spinal anaesthesia (or, much more rarely, with hypnosis or acupuncture).
- Your partner could be present at the birth, could watch the birth through the observation window or could wait outside.
- Your partner, or a midwife, could take photographs of your baby being born, and of her first moments of life, if you wish.
- You could even make a video of the birth.
- If you have regional anaesthesia, you could have music of your choice playing during the birth.
- The medical team caring for you during the birth could give you a running commentary on the operation, telling you what they are doing at each particular point, or they could talk about other matters to take your mind off the operation.
- You and your partner could watch the operation itself, with the help of a mirror if necessary, or you could decide not to.
- If you have general anaesthesia, and your partner is not present, a midwife or another person who was there could recount and describe the birth and the first moments of your baby's life to you when you wake up, if you wish.
- Your baby could be wrapped in a blanket or placed under a heat lamp to keep warm until you wake up or he could be dressed ready to meet you if you prefer.
- Your baby could be washed while you are unconscious so that she is all clean when you wake up or she could be just wiped over so that she is in her nearly newborn state when you first meet her.
- You could be shown your placenta when you wake up, if you so wish.

- You could wake to find your baby in the cot next to your bed, in your partner's arms or snuggled up in bed with you.
- You and your partner could have some time alone with your new baby after the birth.
- You could breastfeed your baby while still in the operating theatre (this is even possible, with help, if you are under general anaesthetic) or in the recovery room, or you could wait until you are on the maternity ward and feel ready to offer him his first feed.
- You could have a single room for the whole of your hospital stay, you could have a single room at first and then transfer to a shared ward or you could be in a shared ward for the entire stay.
- During your hospital stay your baby could sleep in bed with you, could sleep in her cot next to your bed or could be cared for in the nursery while you sleep.
- You could carry out most of the tasks involved in caring for your baby yourself, from early on, or the ward staff could help you look after her until you feel rested and well enough to do so yourself.
- You could receive a full regimen of pain medication during the post-operative period or you could receive only mild painkillers, or you could decline them altogether if you experience little pain or prefer not to take pain relief medication.
- You could be discharged from hospital after just a few days or you could remain in hospital for ten days or more.

EVERY CAESAREAN A GOOD CAESAREAN

The type and quality of care women receive can have an enormous effect on their experience of caesarean childbirth. Whilst we, as caesarean mothers, can press for alternatives that meet our needs and improve our childbirth experiences, there is much that remains out of our hands. It is those who provide our maternity care who have perhaps the most power to shape the caesarean birth experience. It is therefore imperative that health professionals examine the type and quality of care they offer.

What follows are some ideas and suggestions for improving the care of women who give birth by caesarean. I do not offer these as definitive statements, but rather as provisional guidelines for good practice and as a stimulus for further discussion. Some hospitals and practitioners already provide care along these lines, but many do not.

If you have read the preceding chapters of this book, it will be apparent that there are many things that influence the way women feel about giving birth by caesarean. These include the extent of antenatal preparation; whether the caesarean was carried out as an emergency or elective procedure; the type of anaesthesia used; whether complications arose; whether or not the caesarean was perceived to have been necessary and unavoidable; the extent to which the woman was involved in decisions about her maternity care; and the amount of support received before, during and after the birth. In most of these areas there is much that hospitals and health professionals can do to minimise the negative aspects of caesarean birth and to help to make every caesarean a good caesarean.

Firstly, there appears to be a great and presently unmet need for antenatal preparation. The majority of first-time caesarean mothers feel unprepared for caesarean birth.[27] It is recommended that all antenatal classes and childbirth literature should cover caesarean birth, and include some discussion of its medical, practical and emotional aspects. The aim should be to give a realistic awareness of the likelihood of a caesarean being necessary, and of what is involved. By offering such information to all pregnant women, this will help to minimise the distress and sense of shock that often follows an emergency cacsarean birth. Furthermore, when there are indications during pregnancy or labour that a caesarean is likely, or when an elective caesarean is planned, the woman and her partner will need detailed information on caesarean birth, and perhaps several opportunities to ask questions.

There also appear to be strong grounds for encouraging the use of regional anaesthesia for caesarean deliveries. Unless an emergency situation arises in which there is no time to administer regional anaesthesia, or if regional anaesthesia is inadvisable for medical reasons, all women should be offered the opportunity to witness and participate in the birth of their baby. It is important to recognise, however, that a significant proportion of women will choose general anaesthesia and this will be the right decision for them. This decision should be respected and no one should be put under pressure to have regional anaesthesia.

There are a number of things that can be done to minimise the sense of loss — of missing the birth and not sharing the first moments of the baby's life — that is common after a caesarean under general anaesthetic. Something that a significant proportion of couples whose baby is born by general anaesthetic caesarean would appreciate is for the baby's father to be present at the birth. All hospitals might usefully consider reviewing current policies that exclude partners from the operating theatre when general anaesthesia is used. When the partner is not present, for not all couples will want him to be, the couple should be provided with a photograph of their baby being born, if they so wish. In addition, it is very helpful if someone who was present recounts the birth to the parents, telling them what the baby looked like when she was born, her first reactions, when or whether she cried and all that happened to her just after the birth. Some caesarean mothers would also appreciate the opportunity to see the baby in her near-newborn state, before she has been washed and dressed.

It is clear from my research that anaesthetic failure, wound infections and other complications arising during or after a caesarean can be very distressing. It is therefore essential that steps are taken to minimise the occurrence of complications. When complications do arise a woman should be offered an acknowledgement of what has happened to her, an explanation of why the complication occurred and information about any long-term effects and the likelihood of recurrence in a future caesarean.

A caesarean delivery is particularly hard to bear when it is perceived to have been unnecessary or avoidable. It is therefore essential that all medical professionals take a careful and detailed look at their caesarean section rates. Current practices need to be reviewed and the medical evidence scrutinised with a view to halting the seemingly inexorable rise in caesareans. There is also scope for actually reducing the number of caesareans carried out, so that rates settle at a level where all caesareans are of proven benefit to mother and baby.

As well as ensuring that every caesarean is a necessary caesarean, it is also vitally important caesarean mothers receive a full explanation of why their baby needed to be born by caesarean. Often explanations will need to be repeated, and ideally women should receive them when the decision to deliver by caesarean is made, on discharge from hospital and at the six-week check-up, with the opportunity for further contact with the hospital should further explanation be necessary. Caesarean mothers also need information about the likely management of future deliveries.

Something else that has an important influence on the way caesarean birth is experienced is the extent to which women are involved in decision-making — about the management of labour, about alternatives in caesarean birth (see list above) and about the decision to carry out a caesarean. It can make such a difference when women's views and needs are taken into account, when women are offered choices where alternative courses of action are possible and when procedures are carried out only with a woman's informed consent. Then caesarean mothers experience a sense of involvement, participation and control, rather than feeling disempowered or even violated. It is important to be honest with women about situations where obstetric opinions differ or where there is not enough medical research to know what is the best option. Of course, not all women will want to be involved in some of the more medical decisions, but even then it is far preferable to say, for example, 'The medical evidence suggests that in your situation it would be safer to have your baby by caesarean for the following reasons . . . what do you feel about this?', rather than simply 'You've got to have a caesarean'.

The final factor that plays a crucial role in shaping the caesarean experience is the amount of care and support a woman receives before, during and after the birth. When the decision to carry out a caesarean is made it is vital that this is handled with sensitivity and an awareness of the woman's emotional as well as medical needs. The news that a caesarean is necessary is very distressing for some women and they will need time to assimilate this information. For a number of the women in my research, the caesarean was the culmination of a highly distressing labour, and their feelings about having a caesarean are bound up with feelings about events in labour. This is particularly so for women who felt that their caesareans were a consequence of a lack of care during labour, of being in an unsupportive or even hostile environment, or of inappropriate interventions that altered the natural course of labour. So, care and support during labour are very important if all caesarean mothers are to feel positive about their experience. The period just before a caesarean is carried out can also be a very difficult time when many parents feel apprehensive or frightened. The right kind of support and reassurance at this time can help enormously.

Caesarean parents also need support during the birth itself. If regional anaesthesia is being used every effort should be made to put the parents at their ease, to include them in conversations and to remember at all times that this is not just an operation, it is also the birth of a baby. Some parents will want to be told what is happening at each stage during the operation, some will appreciate distracting chat and others will enjoy listening to music during the birth. Once the baby is born the mother should be allowed and encouraged to cuddle her newborn and to breastfeed him if she wishes, whilst the operation is being completed. The baby should not be whisked off to be checked, weighed and cleaned — all this can and should be done at the mother's side.

The parents whose baby is born under general anaesthetic also need care and support. If the baby's father is not present at the birth, and if staffing levels allow, a midwife should stay with him during the seemingly long and often difficult wait until the baby is born. If all is well, the baby should be given to her father to hold and greet just minutes after the birth. The baby's mother should meet her new baby as soon as she regains consciousness, and many will appreciate waking to find the baby in bed with them. Like any other family, caesarean parents will invariably appreciate having some private time alone with their newborn soon after the birth.

All separations should be minimised. In the few hospitals that still routinely put all caesarean babies in special care for a period of observation, this practice should be abandoned. When there is a medical reason why a baby needs special care the parents should be kept fully informed about why this is necessary and about the baby's condition. They should be given a photograph of the baby, and should be taken to see him as soon as possible. A number of caesarean mothers whose babies needed special care were upset that other relatives saw the baby before they did, and hospitals might consider not allowing relatives, other than the baby's father, to see the baby until the mother herself has done so. The time that parents spend with their baby in special care should not be restricted and parents should be encouraged to become involved in the baby's care.

Caesarean mothers also need a lot of care and support during their stay in hospital. This support includes adequate pain relief; practical support with activities like getting out of bed, picking up the baby, walking and washing; and help in caring for the baby, in changing her nappy, dressing and feeding her. There appears to be a particular need for more help with breastfeeding after a caesarean. Women need to be told to press their buzzers whenever they need help, and that the buzzer is not just for emergencies. Staff need to be flexible since caesarean mothers vary in the amount and type of support they need, and needs vary over time as women recover from the operation. Policies also need to be flexible. Some caesarean mothers will appreciate having a single room, particularly in the first few days, others will be happy to be in a shared ward. Some women will appreciate having their babies with them at all times, others would like their babies to be cared for in the nursery at night. Hospitals also need to be flexible about when to discharge caesarean mothers since there is a large variation in the amount of time women want and need to spend in hospital.

Caesarean mothers often need emotional as well as practical support during the postnatal period, and hospitals should endeavour to meet this need. What many mothers would appreciate is for a midwife to be able to sit with them, to listen while they talk through the birth experience, to answer any questions they may have and to acknowledge and legitimate their feelings. There may also be a role for more formal emotional care or therapy, since at least one study has found this to be beneficial.[28]

The type of practical and emotional care outlined here may

appear somewhat Utopian given the current resourcing and staff levels within the health service, but it is nevertheless important to discuss and envisage the sort of care that caesarean mothers need to know what to aim for.

The care and support a caesarean mother needs does not end when she is discharged from hospital. Good and thorough aftercare by the community midwife, GP and health visitor is also very important. These practitioners have a role to play in the emotional as well as medical recovery of caesarean mothers. However, it is vital that practitioners do not assume that all caesarean mothers will inevitably be distressed or depressed about having given birth by caesarean. This is clearly not always the case. They should also be aware that feelings change over time, and that a woman may have many complex and conflicting emotions about the birth. The only way to find out how a woman feels about her caesarean experience is to ask her and listen carefully to her reply. By the very act of listening, by talking with sensitivity and awareness, and by acknowledging the feelings and emotions that arise, practitioners can help women to come to terms with their experience of caesarean childbirth and its emotional aftermath.

I began this book with the words of one caesarean mother who described us as 'the growing and forgotten band of childbearers'. This book is offered as a testament to all caesarean mothers, to speak of and record our experiences in all their diversity, and to make our needs known so that we, and our experiences, are no longer ignored, dismissed or forgotten.

Notes

Introduction

1. Others, e.g. Oakley, Ann & Richards, Martin, 'Women's Experiences of Caesarean Delivery' in Garcia, Jo, Kilpatrick, Robert & Richards, Martin (eds), *The Politics of Maternity Care*, Oxford, Oxford University Press, 1990, p. 183, have also noted the relative lack of research on the social and psychological consequences of caesarean birth.

2. Oakley, Ann, *Women Confined: Towards a Sociology of Childbirth*, Oxford, Martin Robertson, 1980, p. 231.

3. See, for example, Wallace, L., 'Psychological Preparation as a Method of Reducing the Stress of Surgery' in *Journal of Human Stress*, Summer, 1984, pp. 62—77.

Chapter 1: Why a Caesarean?

1. This figure is calculated assuming the following caesarean section rates, which are the figures for 1985 and 1988 respectively, the latest years available: England and Wales — 11.6 per cent, from Francome, Colin, *Changing Childbirth: Interventions in Labour in England and Wales*, London, Maternity Alliance, 1989, p. 9 (data from the Maternity Hospital In-Patient Enquiry and Hospital Activity Analysis gives a figure of 10.6 per cent for England and Wales, but this is thought to be a low estimate, see Francome, op. cit., p. 7); and Scotland — 13.8 per cent, from Donnithorne, Patricia, 'Selected Maternity Statistics' in *New Generation*, vol. 9, no. 4, 1990, p. 15, which gives a figure of 11.8 per cent for Britain as a whole.

2. Payer, Lynn, *Medicine and Culture*, London, Gollancz, 1989, p. 130; Maternity Alliance, *One Birth in Nine*, London, Maternity Alliance, p. 23.

3. Russell, J.G.B., 'Moulding of the Pelvic Outlet' in *Journal of Obstetrics and Gynaecology of the British Commonwealth*, vol. 76, 1969, pp. 817—20.

4. Mahmood, T.A., Campbell, D.M. & Wilson, A.W., 'Maternal Height, Shoe Size and Outcome of labour in White Primigravidas' in *British Medical Journal*, vol. 297, 1988, pp. 515—17.

5. ibid.

6. Enkin, Murray, Keirse, Marc J.N.C. & Chalmers, Iain, *A Guide to Effective Care in Pregnancy and Childbirth*, Oxford, Oxford University Press, 1989, p. 67. This book reports the results of a systematic review

of the effects of various forms of medical care during pregnancy and childbirth. The authors reviewed over 60 journals from the 1950 issues onwards. They also wrote to over 40,000 obstetricians and paediatricians in 18 countries to identify unpublished studies. It is therefore a very useful and authoritative book, whose findings I have drawn upon frequently, along with those in the more comprehensive version of the book, Chalmers, Iain, Enkin, Murray & Keirse, Marc J.N.C. (eds), *Effective Care in Pregnancy and Childbirth*, Oxford, Oxford University Press, 1989.

7. ibid., p. 68.

8. ibid., p. 207.

9. Naaktgeboren, Cornelis, 'The Biology of Childbirth' in Chalmers et al., op. cit., pp. 795–804.

10. Balaskas, Janet, *New Active Birth: A Concise Guide to Natural Childbirth*, London, Thorsons, 1989, p. 10.

11. Ghosh, A., 'Oxytocic Agents and Neonatal Morbidity' in the *Lancet*, vol. 1, 1975, p. 453.

12. Duff, P. et al., 'Management of Premature Rupture of Membranes on Unfavourable Cervix in Term Pregnancy' in *Obstetrics and Gynecology*, vol. 63, 1984, p. 69.

13. Studd, J.W.W. et al., 'The Effect of Lumbar Epidural Analgesia on the Rate of Cervical Dilatation and the Outcome of Labour of Spontaneous Onset' in *British Journal of Obstetrics and Gynaecology*, vol. 87, 1980, pp. 1015–21.

14. Chamberlain, Geoffrey, *Lecture Notes on Obstetrics*, 5th edition, Oxford, Blackwell, 1984, p. 149.

15. Inch, Sally, *Birthrights: A Parents' Guide to Modern Childbirth*, 2nd edition, London, Green Print, 1989, p. 85.

16. Ghosh, op. cit.

17. Balaskas, op. cit., p. 12.

18. Inch, op. cit., p. 115.

19. Enkin et al., op. cit., p. 69; Collea, J.V., Chein, C. & Quilligan, E.J., 'The Randomised Management of Term Frank Breech Presentation' in *American Journal of Obstetrics and Gynecology*, vol. 137, 1980, pp. 235–42.

20. Odent, Michel, 'Natural Protocol for Breech Birth' in Richards, Lynn Baptisti (ed.), *The Vaginal Birth after Cesarean Experience: Birth Stories by Parents and Professionals*, Mass, USA, Bergin & Garvey, p. 202.

21. Enkin et al., op. cit., p. 73.

22. ibid., p. 250.

23. Enkin, Murray, 'Labour and Delivery Following Previous Caesarean Section' in Chalmers et al., op. cit., 1989, p. 1205, cites five such studies.

24. Fairweather, Denys, 'Caesarean Section for Delivery of Very Low Birthweight Babies' in Maternity Alliance, op. cit., London, Maternity Alliance, 1986, pp. 47–50.

25. Enkin et al., op. cit., p. 293.

26. Botting, Beverely, McFarlane, Alison & Price, Frances, *Three, Four and More: A Study of Triplets and Higher Order Births*, London, HMSO, 1990.

27. Payer, op. cit., p. 130.

28. Janowitz, B. et al., 'Cesarean Section in Brazil' in *Social Science and Medicine*, vol. 16, 1982, pp. 19—25.

29. Maternity Alliance, op. cit., 1986, p. 23.

30. Richards, T., 'European Contrasts in Obstetrics' in *British Medical Journal*, vol. 294, 1987, p. 990.

31. Francome, op. cit., 1989, p. 12.

32. Philipp, Elliot, *Caesareans: An Explanation and Preparation*, London, Sidgwick and Jackson, 1988, p. xxvii.

33. Maternity Alliance, op. cit., 1986, p. 19.

34. Payer, op. cit., p. 130.

35. Francome, Colin & Huntingford, Peter J., 'Births by Cesarean-Section in the United States and in Britain' in *Journal of Biosocial Science*, vol. 12, 1980, pp. 353—62.

36. Savage, Wendy, 'Commentary' in Francome, op. cit., 1989, p. 56.

37. Enkin et al., op. cit., 1989, p. 256.

38. Lomas, Jonathan & Enkin, Murray, 'Variations in Operative Delivery Rates' in Chalmers et al., op. cit., 1989, p. 1193.

39. Francome, op. cit., 1989, p. 37.

40. This figure is calculated on the assumption that there are approximately 754,400 births in Britain, around 11.8 per cent of which are by caesarean, and assuming an ideal caesarean rate of around 7 per cent. My assertion that there may be as many as 35,000 unnecessary or avoidable caesareans carried out in Britain every year is similar to research by Professor Richard Lilford and colleagues who found that 30 per cent of caesarean births were unnecessary, as reported in the *Independent,* 31 August, 1990.

41. Reeves, Phil, 'Patients "Given Operations to Avoid Claims"' in the *Independent*, 12 June, 1989.

42. Maternity Alliance, op. cit., 1986, p. 8.

43. Quoted in Francome, op. cit., 1989, p. 32.

44. Bateman, D.E.R., 'Holding Back the Tide of Caesareans' in letter to *British Medical Journal*, vol. 297, 1988, p. 1128.

45. Lomas, Jonathan, 'Holding Back the Tide of Caesareans' in *British Medical Journal*, vol. 297, 1988, pp. 569—70.

46. Quoted in Hodgkinson, Neville, 'Surge in "needless" births by caesarian' in the *Sunday Times*, 9 October, 1988.

47. Maternity Alliance, op. cit., 1986, p. 13.

48. Savage in Francome, op. cit., 1989, p. 56.

49. Maternity Alliance, op. cit., 1986, p. 13.

50. Payer, op. cit., p. 24.

51. Chalmers, I. & Richards, M., 'Intervention and Causal Inference in Obstetric Practice' in T. Chard & M. Richards (eds), *Benefits and*

Hazards of the New Obstetrics, London, Heinemann, 1977.

52. Keirse, Marc J.N.C., 'Augmentation of Labour' in Chalmers et al., op. cit., 1989, p. 958.

53. Renfew, Mary, 'Commentary' in Francome, op. cit., 1989, p. 53.

54. Inch, op. cit., p. 36.

55. Enkin et al., op. cit., p. 192.

56. Inch, op. cit., p. 90.

57. Enkin et al., op. cit., p. 193.

58. Savage, Wendy, *A Savage Enquiry: Who Controls Childbirth?*, London, Virago, 1986, p. 88.

59. Enkin et al., op. cit., 1989, p. 203.

60. Kitzinger, Sheila, *Freedom and Choice in Childbirth*, Harmondsworth, Penguin, 1987, p. 253.

61. Arms, Suzanne, *The Immaculate Deception*, Boston, Houghton Mifflin, 1975; Rich, Adrienne, *Of Woman Born*, London, Virago, 1977.

62. Quoted in 'Caesarean Controversy' in the *Independent*, 28 August.

63. Brooks, Melissa, *Caesarean Birth: A Guide for Parents*, London, Optima, 1989, p. 12.

Chapter 2: The Easy Way to Have a Baby?

1. Prendergast, Shirley & Prout, Alan, 'Learning about Birth: Parenthood and Sex Education in English Secondary Schools' in Garcia, Jo, Kilpatrick, Robert & Richards, Martin (eds), *The Politics of Maternity Care*, Oxford, Oxford University Press, pp. 137–8.

2. ibid., p. 139.

3. Knight, Angela, 'Giving Birth by Caesarean' in *Mother and Baby*, May, 1990.

4. Nancy Kohner, *Pregnancy Book*, London, Health Education Authority, 1988, p. 54.

5. For example, Stoppard, Miriam, *The Baby and Co Pregnancy and Birth Handbook*, London, Dorling Kindersley, 1986.

6. For example, Kitzinger, Sheila, *The Experience of Childbirth*, London, Gollancz, 1972.

7. Nash, Barbara, *The Complete Book of Babycare*, London, Octopus Books, 1978, p. 101.

8. Savage, Wendy, *A Savage Enquiry: Who Controls Childbirth?*, London, Virago, 1986, p. 84.

9. For example, obstetrician Anthony Kenney quoted in Read, Cathy, 'Hard Labour, Sweet Deliverance' in the *Independent* on Sunday, 16 September, 1990. Other obstetricians — Feldman, G.B. & Freiman, J.A., 'Prohylactic Cesarean Section at Term?' in *New England Journal of Medicine*, vol. 312, 1985, pp. 1264–67 — have seriously recommended offering elective caesareans to all pregnant women.

10. Hall, Marion, H., 'When a Woman Asks for a Caesarean Section' in *British Medical Journal*, vol. 294, 1987, p. 201.

11. Rubin, G.L., Paterson, H.B., Rochat, R.W., McCarthy, B.J. &

Terry, J.S., 'Maternal Death after Cesarean Section in Georgia' in *American Journal of Obstetrics and Gynecology*, vol. 139, 1981, pp. 681—5.

12. Enkin, Murray, Keirse, Marc J.N.C. & Chalmers, Iain, *A Guide to Effective Care in Pregnancy and Childbirth*, Oxford, Oxford University Press, 1989, p. 249.

13. Enkin et al., op. cit., p. 259.

14. Shearer, Madeleine, cited in Cohen, Nancy Wainer & Estner, Lois J., *Silent Knife: Cesarean Prevention and Vaginal Birth after Cesarean*, Mass, USA, Bergin & Garvey, 1983, p. 31.

15. Hurry, D.J., Larsen, B. & Charles, D., 'Effects of Postcesarean Section Febrile Morbidity on Subsequent Fertility' in *Obstetrics & Gynecology*, vol. 64, 1984, pp. 256—60; Hemminki, E., Graubord, B.I., Hoffman, H.J., Mosher, W.D. & Fetterly, K., 'Caesarean Section and Subsequent Fertility' in *Fertility and Sterility*, vol. 43, pp. 250—8.

16. Hurst, Martha & Summey, Pamela, S., 'Childbirth and Social Class' in *Social Science and Medicine*, vol. 18, 1983, pp. 621—31.

17. Kitzinger, Sheila, *Freedom and Choice in Childbirth*, Harmondsworth, Penguin, 1987, p. 254.

18. Enkin et al., op. cit., p. 249.

Chapter 3: Born a Cut Above

1. Lomas, Jonathan & Enkin, Murray, 'Variations in Operative Delivery Rates' in Chalmers, Iain, Enkin, Murray & Keirse, Marc J.N.C. (eds), *Effective Care in Pregnancy and Childbirth*, vol. 2, Oxford, Oxford University Press, 1989, p. 1192.

2. Molloy, B.G., Sheil, O. & Duigan, N.M., 'Delivery after Caesarean Section: Review of 2176 consecutive cases' in *British Medical Journal*, vol. 294, 1987, pp. 1645—7.

3. Pearson, Jim & Rees, Gareth, 'Technique of Caesarean Section' in Chalmers et al., op. cit., p. 1239.

4. Inch, Sally, *Birthrights: A Parents' Guide to Modern Childbirth*, 2nd edition, London, Green Print, 1989, p. 112.

5. Enkin, Murray, Keirse, Marc J.N.C. & Chalmers, Iain, *A Guide to Effective Care in Pregnancy and Childbirth*, Oxford, Oxford University Press, 1989, p. 290.

6. Clement, Sarah, 'Caesarean Childbirth: What are its Psychological Effects?', unpublished paper. In this paper I present the results of an analysis of 120 questionnaires completed by caesarean mothers recruited via *Practical Parenting* magazine. The sample, being self-selected, cannot tell us about caesarean mothers in general but can provide important information about differences within this group, and gives some answers to the question 'What makes a caesarean a positive or a negative experience?'.

7. ibid.

8. Study cited in Philipp, Elliot, *Caesareans: An Explanation and Preparation*, London, Sidgwick and Jackson, 1988, p. 122.

9. Clement, op. cit.

10. Hodgkinson, Neville, 'Nightmares in Surgery' in the *Sunday Times*, 25 June, 1989.

11. ibid.

12. Professor James Payne speaking on 'Awake and in Pain' on *Taking Liberties*, BBC2, 28 March, 1989.

13. David Jessel speaking on 'Awake and in Pain'.

14. Melville, Joy, 'When Pain Springs a Trap' in the *Sunday Times*, 19 March, 1989; Hodgkinson, op. cit.

15. Beech, Beverley Lawrence, *Who's Having your Baby? A Health Rights Handbook for Maternity Care*, London, Camden Press, 1987, p. 93.

16. Cohen, Nancy Wainer & Estner, Lois J., *Silent Knife: Cesarean Prevention and Vaginal Birth After Cesarean*, Mass, USA, Bergin & Garvey, 1983, p. 32.

17. Jordan, Michael, J., 'Anaesthesia' in Philipp, op. cit., p. 89.

18. Clement, op. cit.

19. ibid.

20. ibid.; also Cranley, M.S., Hedahl, K.J. & Pegg, S.H., 'Women's Perceptions of Vaginal and Cesarean Deliveries' in *Nursing Research*, vol. 32, 1983, pp. 10—15.

21. Kitzinger, Sheila, *Freedom and Choice in Childbirth*, Harmondsworth, Penguin, 1987, p. 273.

22. Beech, op. cit., p. 68.

23. Rhoden, N.K., 'The Judge in the Delivery Room: The Emergence of Court-Ordered Cesareans' in *California Law Review*, vol. 74, 1986, pp. 1951—2030.

24. Enkin et al., op. cit., p. 363.

25. Philipp, op. cit., p. 122.

26. Clement, op. cit.

27. ibid.

Chapter 4: Early Days

1. Clement, Sarah, 'Caesarean Childbirth: What are its Psychological Effects?', unpublished paper, 1990.

2. ibid.

3. Hall, Marion, 'Crisis in the Maternity Services' in *British Medical Journal*, vol. 297, 1988, pp. 500—1.

4. This was apparent in my own research. Other research — Moss, Peter, Bolland, Gill, Foxman, Ruth & Owen, Charlie, 'The Hospital Inpatient Stay: The Experience of First-time Parents' in *Child: Care, Health and Development*, vol. 13, 1987, pp. 153—67 — reports that women who had had caesarean births were more dissatisfied with their hospital stay than other women.

5. Clement, op. cit.

6. Hunt, Liz, 'Patients "Suffering Unnecessary pain After Surgery"' in the *Independent*, 26 September, 1990.

7. ibid.

8. Levy, V., 'The Maternity Blues in Post-partum and Post-operative Women' in *British Journal of Psychiatry*, vol. 151, 1987, pp. 368—72.

9. Yalom, I.D., Lunde, D.T., Moos, R.H. & Hamburg, D.A., 'Postpartum Blues Syndrome' in *Archives of General Psychiatry*, vol. 18, 1968, pp. 16—27.

10. Levy, op. cit.

11. Ellis, Brian, W., 'Surgical Blues' in the *Independent*, 15 September, 1987.

12. Beech, Beverley Lawrence, *Who's Having your Baby? A Health Rights Handbook for Maternity Care*, London, Camden Press, 1987, p. 71.

13. Adams, J., Hayes, J. & Hopson, B., *Transition: Understanding and Managing Personal Change*, Oxford, Martin Robertson, 1976.

14. Panuthos, Claudia & Romeo, Catherine, *Ended Beginnings: Healing Childbearing Losses*, Mass, USA, Bergin & Garvey, 1984, p. 137.

Chapter 5: The Wound in the Mind

1. Line from the poem 'Once a Cesarean — Now What?' by Jami Osborne, in Cohen, Nancy Wainer & Estner, Lois J., *Silent Knife: Cesarean Prevention and Vaginal Birth after Cesarean*, Mass, USA, Bergin & Garvey, 1983, p. 56.

2. Cranley, M.S., Hedahl, K.J. & Pegg, S.H., 'Women's Perceptions of Vaginal and Cesarean Deliveries' in *Nursing Research*, vol. 32, 1983, pp. 10—15; Garel, M., Lelong, N. & Kaminski, M., 'Psychological Consequences of Caesarean Childbirth in Primiparas' in *Journal of Psychosomatic Obstetrics and Gynaecology*, vol. 6, 1987, pp. 197—209; Clement, Sarah, 'Caesarean Childbirth: What are its Psychological Effects?', unpublished paper.

3. Cranley et al., op. cit.; Garel et al., op. cit.

4. Clement, op. cit.

5. Hall, Joan Joffe 'A Labor-saving Device' in Ashford, Janet Isaacs (ed.), *Birth Stories: The Experience Remembered*, San Francisco, The Crossing Press, 1984, p. 23.

6. Cohen & Estner, op. cit., p. 225.

7. ibid., p. 40.

8. This point was first made by Cohen & Estner, op. cit., p. 4.

9. Richards, Lynn Baptisti, *The Vaginal Birth After Cesarean Experience: Birth Stories by Parents and Professionals*, Mass, USA, Bergin & Garvey, 1987, pp. 119, 189; Cohen & Estner, op. cit., pp. 98—9.

10. I have borrowed this phrase from the title of a chapter in Oakley, Ann, *Telling the Truth about Jerusalem*, Oxford, Basil Blackwell, 1986, pp. 14—17.

11. Price, Jane, *Motherhood: What it Does to Your Mind*, London, Pandora Press, 1988, p. 41.

12. Flint, Caroline, quoted in Raphael-Leff, Joan, *Psychological Processes of Childbearing*, London, Chapman & Hall, 1991, p. 301.

13. Atwood, Margaret, *Bodily Harm*, London, Virago, 1983, p. 23.

14. Kitzinger, Sheila, 'When Giving Birth Feels Degrading' in the *Independent*, 29 August, 1989.

15. Stewart, Nancy, 'Obstetric Drugs and Technology' in Claxton, Ros (ed.), *Birth Matters: Issues and Alternatives in Childbirth*, London, Unwin Paperbacks, 1986, p. 37.

16. Raphael-Leff, op. cit., p. 250.

17. Fisch, Robert & colleagues, quoted in 'Long-term Effects of Catastrophe' in the *Independent*, 12 November, 1989.

18. Melville, Joy, 'Tackling Postnatal Depression' in the *Sunday Times*, 25 June, 1989.

19. For example, Bradley, C.F., Ross, S.E. & Warnyca, J., 'A Prospective Study of Mothers' Attitudes and Feelings Following Cesarean and Vaginal Births' in *Birth: Issues in Perinatal Care and Education*, vol. 10, 1983, pp. 79–83; Padawer, J.A., Fagan, C., Janoff-Bulman, R. & Strickland, B.R., 'Women's Psychological Adjustment Following Emergency Cesarean Versus Vaginal Delivery' in *Psychology of Women Quarterly*, vol. 12, 1988, pp. 25–34.

20. For example, Kendall, R.E. et al., 'The Social and Obstetric Correlates of Psychiatric Admission in the Puerperium' in *Psychological Medicine*, vol. 11, 1981, pp. 341–50; Gottlieb, Susan E. & Barrett, David E., 'Effects of Unanticipated Cesarean Section on Mothers, Infants and their Interaction in the First Months of Life' in *Journal of Developmental and Behavioral Pediatrics*, vol. 7, 1986, pp. 180–185; Garel et al., op. cit.

21. Clement, op. cit.

22. Panuthos, Claudia & Bierkoe-Peer, Barbara, *The Emotional Ups and Downs of Childbirth*, Boston, People Place, 1981.

Chapter 6: Mother and Child

1. Steele, M., Moltz, H. & Rowland, D., 'Adrenal Disruption of Maternal Behavior in the Cesarean-sectioned Rat' in *Hormones and Behavior*, vol. 7, 1976, pp. 473–9; Alexander, G., Stevens, D. & Bradley, L.R., 'Maternal Behaviour in Ewes following Cesarean Section' in *Applied Animal Behavioural Science*, vol. 19, 1988, pp. 273–7.

2. Pederson, F.A., Zaslow, M.J., Cain, R.L. & Anderson, B.J., 'Cesarean Childbirth: Psychological Implications for Mothers and Fathers' in *Infant Mental Health Journal*, vol. 2, 1981, pp. 257–63; Trowell, Judith, 'Possible Effects of Emergency Cesarean-section on the Mother-child Relationship' in *Early Human Development*, vol. 7, 1982, pp. 41–51.

3. Garel, M., Lelong, N. & Kaminski, M., 'Follow-up Study of Psychological Consequences of Cesarean Childbirth' in *Early Human Development*, vol. 16, 1988, pp. 271–82.

4. Bradley, Christine, F., Ross, Susan E. & Warnyca, Jennifer, 'A Prospective Study of Mothers' Attitudes and Feelings Following

Cesarean and Vaginal Births' in *Birth: Issues in Perinatal Care & Education*, vol. 10, 1983, pp. 79—83.

5. Field, Tiffany, M. & Widmayer, Susan, M., 'Developmental Follow-up of Infants Delivered by Cesarean Section and General Anesthesia' in *Infant Behavior & Development*, vol. 3, 1980, pp. 253—64.

6. Tulman, Lorraine, J., 'Initial Handling of Newborn Infants by Vaginally and Cesarean-delivered Mothers' in *Nursing Research*, vol. 35, 1986, pp. 296—300; Hwang, Carl. P., 'Cesarean Childbirth in Sweden: Effects on the Mother and Father-infant Relationship' in *Infant Mental Health Journal*, vol. 8, 1987, pp. 91—9.

7. Clement, Sarah, 'Caesarean Childbirth: What are its Psychological Effects?', unpublished paper, 1990.

8. Robson, Kay, M. & Kumar, R., 'Delayed Onset of Maternal Affection after Childbirth' in *British Journal of Psychiatry*, vol. 136, 1980, pp. 347—53.

9. MacFarlane, J.A., Smith, D.M. & Garrow, D.H., 'The Relationship between Mother and Neonate' in Kitzinger, S. & Davis, J.A. (eds), *The Place of Birth*, Oxford, Oxford University Press, 1978.

10. Clement, op. cit.

11. ibid.

12. Peterson, Gail H. & Mehl, Lewis E., 'Some Determinants of Maternal Attachment' in *American Journal of Psychiatry*, vol. 135, 1978, pp. 1168—73.

13. Klaus, Marshall H. & Kennell, John H., 'Labor, Birth and Bonding' in Klaus, M.H. & Kennell, J.H. (eds), *Parent-Infant Bonding*, St Louis, Missouri, Mosby, 1982, p. 39.

14. ibid., p. 55.

15. Kitzinger, Sheila, *Women as Mothers*, London, Fontana, 1978, p. 192.

16. Klaus & Kennel, op. cit., p. 92.

17. Clement, op. cit.

18. ibid.

19. Raphael-Leff, Joan , *Psychological Processes of Childbearing*, London, Chapman & Hall, 1991, p. 446.

20. Cramer, Bertrand, cited in Kennell John, H. & Klaus, Marshall H., 'Caring for the Parents of Premature or Sick Infants' in Klaus & Kennell, op. cit., 1982.

21. Reader, Fran & Savage, Wendy, *Coping with Caesarean and Other Difficult Births*, Edinburgh, MacDonald, 1983, p. 80.

22. Raphael-Leff, op. cit., p. 454.

23. Panuthos, Claudia & Romeo, Catherine, *Ended Beginnings: Healing Childbearing Losses*, Mass, USA, Bergin & Garvey, 1984, p. 137.

24. Raphael-Leff, op. cit., p. 455.

25. Panuthos & Romeo, op. cit., p. 38.

26. Martin, J., *Infant Feeding 1975: Attitudes and Practice in England and Wales*, OCPS, Social Survey Division, London, HMSO, 1978.

27. Trowell, op. cit.; study by Victoria, C.G., Huttley, S.R.A. & Baros,

F.C., cited in *New Generation*, vol. 9, no. 3, 1990, p. 32; study by Kearney, M.H. et al., cited in *New Generation*, vol. 9, no. 4, 1990, p. 33.

28. Enkin, Murray, Keirse, Marc J.N.C. & Chalmers, Iain, *A Guide to Effective Care in Pregnancy and Childbirth*, Oxford, Oxford University Press, 1989, p. 314.

29. Hwang, op. cit.

30. National Childbirth Trust, *Breastfeeding after a Caesarean Section*, leaflet, London, NCT, 1990.

31. Enkin et al., op. cit., p. 319.

32. Clement, op. cit.

33. Moss, Peter, Bolland, Gill, Foxman, Ruth & Owen, Charlie, 'The Hospital Inpatient Stay: The Experience of First-time Parents' in *Child: Care, Health and Development*, vol. 13, 1987, pp. 153—67.

34. Lomas, Jonathan & Enkin, Murray, 'Variations in Operative Delivery Rates' in Chalmers, Iain, Enkin, Murray & Keirse, Marc J.N.C., (eds) *Effective Care in Pregnancy and Childbirth*, vol. 2, Oxford, Oxford University Press, 1989, p. 1153.

35. Field & Widmayer, op. cit.

36. Entwisle, Dorris R. & Alexander, Karl L., 'Long-term Effects of Cesarean Delivery on Parents' Beliefs and Children's Schooling' in *Developmental Psychology*, vol. 23, 1987, pp. 676—82.

37. English, Jane Butterfield, *Different Doorway: Adventures of a Caesarean Born*, California, Earth Heart, 1985.

38. Cohen, Nancy Wainer & Estner, Lois, J., *Silent Knife: Cesarean Prevention and Vaginal Birth after Cesarean*, Mass, USA, Bergin & Garvey, 1983, p. 241.

39. Kitzinger, Sheila & Kitzinger, Celia, *Talking with Children about Things that Matter*, London, Pandora Press, 1989, pp. 117—18.

40. Le Sieg, Theo, *Are You my Mother?*, London, HarperCollins, 1968.

41. Bettelheim, Bruno, *A Good Enough Parent*, London, Pan Books, 1987, pp. 139—45.

42. Altman, April, 'From ICU to Empirical Midwifery' in Richards, Lynn Baptisti (ed.), *The Vaginal Birth after Cesarean Experience: Birth Stories by Parents and Professionals*, Mass, USA, Bergin & Garvey, 1987, p. 93.

Chapter 7: Partners' Perspectives

1. Clement, Sarah, 'Caesarean Childbirth: What are its Psychological Effects?', unpublished paper, 1990.

2. Erb, Lois, Hill, Gail & Houston, Doreen, 'A Survey of Parents' Attitudes toward their Cesarean Births in Manitoba Hospitals' in *Birth: Issues in Perinatal Care and Education*, vol. 10, 1983, pp. 85—91; May, Katharyn & Sollid, Deanna T., 'Unanticipated Cesarean Birth from the Father's Perspective' in *Birth: Issues in Perinatal Care and Education*, vol. 11, 1984, pp. 87—95.

3. Consultants' replies were reported in *Newslink* (Newsletter of the Caesarean Support Network), issues 13, 14 & 15, 1989.

4. Huntingford, Peter, *Birth Right,* London, BBC Books, 1985, p. 132.

5. Letter from Sue Johnson in *Newslink* (Newsletter of the Caesarean Support Network), issue 14, 1989, p. 4.

6. Huntingford, op. cit., p. 132.

7. Cranley, M.S., Hedahl, K.J. & Pegg, S.H., 'Women's Perceptions of Vaginal and Cesarean Deliveries' in *Nursing Research,* vol. 32, 1983, pp. 10—15.

8. The father's campaign is detailed in *Newslink* (Newsletter of the Caesarean Support Network), issue 14, 1989.

9. Clement, op. cit.

10. Martin Estner in Cohen, Nancy Wainer & Estner, Lois J., *Silent Knife: Cesarean Prevention and Vaginal Birth after Cesarean*, Mass, USA, Bergin & Garvey, 1983, p. 219.

11. Palkovitz, Rob, 'Father's Birth Attendance, Early Contact, and Extended Contact with their Newborns: A Critical Review' in *Child Development*, vol. 56, 1985, pp. 392—406.

12. Hwang, Carl, P., 'Cesarean Childbirth in Sweden: Effects on the Mother and Father-Infant Relationship' in *Infant Mental Health Journal*, vol. 8, 1985, pp. 91—9.

13. Paul Cohen in Cohen & Estner, op. cit., p. 212.

14. ibid., p. 213.

15. Cohen & Estner, op. cit., p. 272.

Chapter 8: Coming to Terms

1. Clement, Sarah, 'Caesarean Childbirth: What are its Psychological Effects?', unpublished paper, 1990.

2. Cohen, Nancy Wainer & Estner, Lois J., *Silent Knife: Cesarean Prevention and Vaginal Birth after Cesarean,* Mass, USA, Bergin & Garvey, 1983, p. 73.

3. Affonso, Dyanne D., 'Missing Pieces: A Study of Postpartum Feelings' in *Birth and the Family Journal*, vol. 14, 1977, pp. 159—64.

4. Jean Robinson, former Chairwoman of the Patients' Association and lay member of the General Medical Council, quoted in Lloyd, Ann, 'When Patients Find Insult is Being Added to Injury' in the *Independent,* 7 September, 1990.

5. Beech, Beverley Lawrence, *Who's Having Your Baby? A Health Rights Handbook for Maternity Care*, London, Camden Press, 1987, Chpt 9, pp. 106—20.

6. Panuthos, Claudia & Romeo, Catherine, *Ended Beginnings: Healing Childbearing Losses*, Mass, USA, Bergin & Garvey, 1984, p. 150.

Chapter 9: Next Time

1. Hare, John, quoted in Caesarean Support Group of Cambridge, *Caesarean Birth: A Handbook for Parents*, Cambridge, Cambridge Caesarean Support Group, 1988.

2. Cohen, Nancy Wainer & Estner, Lois J., *Silent Knife: Cesarean Prevention and Vaginal Birth after Cesarean*, Mass, USA, Bergin & Garvey, 1983, p. 376.

3. Clement, Sarah, 'Caesarean Childbirth: What are its Psychological Effects?', unpublished paper, 1990.

4. Personal communication with a consultant in a London hospital who claimed to have carried out this seventeenth caesarean.

5. For example, Murray Enkin in Enkin, Murray, 'Labour and Delivery Following Previous Caesarean Section' in Chalmers, Iain, Enkin, Murray & Keirse, Marc J.N.C. (eds), *Effective Care in Pregnancy and Childbirth*, vol. 2, Oxford, Oxford University Press, 1989, pp. 1182—95.

6. Phillip, Elliot, *Caesareans: An Explanation and Preparation*, London, Sidgwick & Jackson, 1988, p. 65.

7. Enkin, Murray, Keirse, Marc J.N.C. & Chalmers, Iain, *A Guide to Effective Care in Pregnancy and Childbirth*, Oxford, Oxford University Press, 1989, p. 250, states that 'The technique of decision analysis has been used to determine the optimal delivery policy after previous caesarean section. The probabilities and utilities of a number of possible outcomes . . . can be put into a mathematical model comparing different policies. Over a wide range of probabilities and utilities, which included all reasonable values, trial of labour proved to be the logical choice.'

8. Davies, Jennifer A. & Spencer, John A.D., 'Trial of Scar' in *British Journal of Hospital Medicine*, vol. 40, 1988, pp. 379—81 reviewed eleven studies on over 4,000 women having trials of labour after a previous caesarean and found an overall vaginal delivery rate of 82 per cent; Enkin, op. cit., p. 1198, also reviewed eleven studies containing over 7,000 women and found a rate of 79 per cent.

9. McClain, Carol S., 'Why Women Choose Trial of Labor or Repeat Cesarean Section' in *Journal of Family Practice*, vol. 21, 1985, pp. 210—16.

10. See, for example, accounts in Kitzinger, Sheila, *Giving Birth: How it Really Feels*, London, Gollancz, 1987, pp. 150—2; *Newslink* (Newsletter of the Caesarean Support Network), issue 8, 1987, pp. 9—10.

11. Richards, Lynn Baptisti, *The Vaginal Birth after Cesarean Experience: Birth Stories by Parents and Professionals*, Mass, USA, Bergin & Garvey, 1987, pp. 43—51.

12. This woman was one case in a study by Browne, A.D.H. & McGrath, J., 'Vaginal Delivery after Previous Caesarean Section' in *Journal of Obstetrics and Gynaecology of the British Commonwealth*, vol. 72, 1965, pp. 557—63.

13. Enkin, op. cit., p. 1205, cites five such studies.

14. ibid., p. 1204.

15. Davies and Spencer, op. cit., combined data from five separate studies and found a vaginal delivery rate of 69 per cent in trials of labour after two or more previous caesareans.

16. In studies reviewed by Cohen & Estner, op. cit., p. 108, rates varied from 1 to 3 per cent, but Cohen & Estner state that they believe the rate to be closer to 1 per cent; Enkin et al., op. cit., p. 251, quotes a figure of 2.2 per cent.

17. Enkin et al., op. cit., p. 251.

18. The study by Browne & McGrath, op. cit., contained twenty-one women having trials of labour with classical scars. Cohen and Estner, op. cit., p. 112, have worked with six such women. In Richards, op. cit., pp. 43—51, there is an account of a woman who gives birth vaginally after two classical and two lower segment caesareans.

19. Dewhurst, C.J., 'The Ruptured Caesarean Section Scar' in *Journal of Obstetrics and Gynaecology of the British Empire*, vol. 64, 1957, pp. 113—18.

20. MacAfee cited in Cohen and Estner, op. cit., p. 109.

21. Levine, Mitch, 'Classical VBAC' in Richards, op. cit., 1987, p. 187.

22. Enkin et al., op. cit., p. 251—2.

23. Davies and Spencer, op. cit.

24. Phelan, J.P., Clark, S.L., Diaz, F. & Paul, R.H., 'Vaginal Birth after Cesarean' in *American Journal of Obstetrics and Gynecology*, vol. 157, 1987, pp. 1510—15.

25. Enkin et al., op. cit., p. 68.

26. Spencer & Davies, op. cit.

27. Cohen and Estner, op. cit., p. 98, cite studies involving ninety-six women who gave birth vaginally after previous caesareans for disproportion, and they themselves have worked with around 100 such women.

28. Cohen and Estner, op. cit., p. 336, have worked with three women who had been told that their pelvis was completely contracted and subsequently gave birth vaginally.

29. Twist, Judy and Allen, 'The Movement Continues' in Richards, op. cit., 1987, p. 108—21.

30. This was the conclusion of the panel of the Canadian Consensus Conference on Aspects of Caesarean Birth, reported in Enkin, op. cit., p. 1212.

31. Cohen & Estner, op. cit., p. 98, state that the majority of the hundred or so women they have worked with who had VBACs after previous caesareans for disproportion gave birth to larger babies. In studies by Silfen & Wilf and Saldana, reported in Cohen & Estner, op. cit., p. 98, eleven and six women respectively, who had had previous caesareans for disproportion had vaginal births with larger babies.

32. Enkin, op. cit., p. 1206.

33. Savage, Wendy, *A Savage Enquiry: Who Controls Childbirth?*, London, Virago, 1986, p. 37.

34. ibid., p. 93.

35. McKinney, Kenneth, 'Mandatory Labor after Previous Cesarean' in Richards, op. cit., 1987, p. 189.

36. Lavin, J.P., Stephens, R.J., Miodovnik, M. & Barden, T.P., 'Vaginal Delivery in Patients with a Previous Cesarean Section' in *Obstetrics and Gynecology*, vol. 59, 1982, p. 135.

37. This was the conclusion of the panel of the Canadian Consensus Conference on Aspects of Caesarean Birth, reported in Enkin, op. cit., p. 1212.

38. Lavin et al., op. cit., cite eighty-three cases of trials of labour with a breech baby; Cohen & Estner, op. cit., p. 101, report two studies containing thirty-two women who had breech vaginal births after a previous caesarean and they themselves have worked with two such women.

39. Williams, Yvonne, 'Vaginal Birth following Caesarean Section' in *AIMS Quarterly Journal*, vol. 2, no. 2, 1990, pp. 18–19.

40. This was the conclusion of the panel of the Canadian Consensus Conference on Aspects of Caesarean Birth, reported in Enkin, op. cit., p. 1212.

41. Cohen and Estner, op. cit., p. 101, cite studies containing seventeen sets of twins born vaginally after a previous caesarean, and have themselves worked with three women who had VBAC twins; Weston, Meg, 'VBAC Triplets' in Richards, op. cit., pp. 51–6.

42. Shearer quoted in Cohen & Estner, op. cit., pp. 101–2.

43. In their review of research on trials of labour after a previous caesarean, Davies & Spencer, op. cit., p. 378, conclude that 'The rate of scar rupture is not affected by factors such as febrile morbidity with the previous caesarean section.'

44. Wilson, quoted in Cohen & Estner, op. cit., p. 100.

45. Williams, op. cit.

46. Beech, Beverley Lawrence, *Who's Having Your Baby? A Health Rights Handbook for Maternity Care*, London, Camden Press, 1987, p. 69.

47. Enkin et al., op. cit., p. 255.

48. Shearer quoted in Cohen & Estner, op. cit., p. 105.

49. Williams, op. cit. See also replies to the Caesarean Support Network's survey in *Newslink* (Newsletter of the Caesarean Support Network), issues 16 and 17/18, 1990.

50. Enkin et al., op.cit., p. 248.

51. Cohen & Estner, op. cit., p. 84.

52. Enkin et al., op. cit., p. 254.

53. Cohen & Estner, op. cit., p. 86.

54. Molloy, B.G., Sheil, O. & Duignan, N.M., 'Delivery after Caesarean Section: Review of 2176 consecutive cases' in *British Medical Journal*, vol. 294, 1987, pp. 1645–7.

55. None of the eight ruptures in the study by Molloy et al., op. cit., was preceeded by pain.

56. Case, B., Corcoran, R., Jeffcoate, N. & Randle, G.H., 'Caesarean Section and its Place in Modern Obstetric Pracice' in *Journal of Obstetrics and Gynaecology of the British Commonwealth*, vol. 78, 1971, pp. 203–14.

57. Shy, K.K., LoGerfo, J.P. & Karp, L.E., 'Evaluation of Elective Repeat Cesarean Section as a Standard of Care: An application of Decision Analysis' in *American Journal of Obstetrics and Gynecology*, vol. 139, 1981, pp. 123–9.

58. Enkin, op. cit., p. 1203.

59. Dewhurst, op. cit.

60. Enkin et al., op. cit., p. 254.

61. Spencer & Davies, op. cit., cite three studies indicating this.

62. Packham, Diane, 'Vaginal Birth after Caesarean Section: Survey by Caesarean Support Network' in *AIMS Quarterly Journal*, vol. 2, no. 4, 1990, p. 10.

63. Reported in Enkin, op. cit., p. 1212.

64. Packham, op. cit.

65. Cohen & Estner, op. cit., p. 84.

66. ibid., p. 162.

67. Packham, op. cit.

68. Enkin et al., op. cit., p. 184.

69. ibid., pp. 184–5.

70. ibid., p. 186.

71. Inch, Sally, *Birthrights: A Parents' Guide to Modern Childbirth*, London, Green Print, 1989, p. 54.

72. Enkin et al., op. cit., p. 262.

73. Salzmann, B., 'Rupture of Low-Segment Cesarean Section Scars' in *Obstetrics and Gynecology*, vol. 23, 1964, p. 460.

74. Molloy, op. cit.

75. Cohen & Estner, p. 266.

76. Enkin et al., op. cit., p. 254.

77. ibid., p. 253.

78. ibid., p. 252.

79. Williams, op. cit.

80. Beech, op. cit., p. 68, states that 'any doctor or midwife giving treatment which the mother has refused leaves him/herself open to a charge of assault'.

81. Cohen & Estner, op. cit., p. 111, have worked with twenty women who had home births after a previous caesarean; there are accounts of ten VBAC home births in Richards, op. cit.; and two in *AIMS Quarterly Journal*, vol. 2, no. 2, 1990, pp. 9–12.

82. Oliver, Barbara, 'Home Birth after Caesarean' in *AIMS Quarterly Journal*, vol. 2., no. 2, 1990, p. 9.

83. Wesson, Nicky, *Home Birth: A Practical Guide*, London, Optima, 1990, pp. 81–2.

84. ibid., p. 86.

85. Clement, op. cit.

86. ibid.; Tcheng, Donna M., 'Emotional Response of Primary and Repeat Cesarean Mothers to the Cesarean Method of Childbirth' in *Health Care for Women International*, vol. 5, 1984, pp. 323–33.

87. Clement, op. cit.

88. These are words used by the VBAC mothers in my research, in Cohen & Estner, op. cit., and in Richards, op. cit.

89. Cohen & Estner, op. cit., p. 70.

Chapter 10: What is to be Done

1. Statistic for 1980, reported in Balaskas, Janet, *New Active Birth: A*

Concise Guide to Natural Childbirth, London, Thorsons, 1989, p. 16.

2. See, for example, Balaskas, ibid.

3. Lomas, Jonathan & Enkin, Murray, 'Variations in Operative Delivery Rates' in Chalmers, Iain, Enkin, Murray & Keirse, Marc J.N.C. (eds), *Effective Care in Pregnancy and Childbirth*, vol. 2, Oxford, Oxford University Press, 1989, p. 1192.

4. Klein, M.C. quoted in Lomas & Enkin, op. cit., 1986, p. 1192.

5. Balaskas, op. cit., p. 177.

6. Kitzinger, Sheila, *Freedom and Choice in Childbirth*, Harmondsworth, Penguin, 1987, p. 200.

7. Balaskas, op. cit., p. 176.

8. Kitzinger, op. cit., p. 201; Balaskas, op. cit., pp. 175—6.

9. Enkin, Murray, Keirse, Marc J.N.C. & Chalmers, Iain, *A Guide to Effective Care in Pregnancy and Childbirth*, Oxford, Oxford University Press, 1989, p. 156.

10. ibid., p. 155.

11. ibid., p. 200.

12. ibid., p. 177.

13. See, for example, James, Jessica, 'On Being a Birth Attendant' in *New Generation*, vol. 9, no. 2, 1990, pp. 22—5.

14. Balaskas, op. cit., pp. 10, 12.

15. ibid., pp. 10—11.

16. Russell, J.G.B., 'Moulding of the Pelvic Outlet' in *Journal of Obstetrics and Gynaecology of the British Commonwealth*, vol. 76, 1969, pp. 817—20.

17. Enkin et al., op. cit., p. 207.

18. ibid., pp. 207—8.

19. Ghosh, A., 'Oxytocic Agents and Neonatal Morbidity' in *Lancet*, vol. 1, 1975, p. 453.

20. Enkin et al., op. cit., pp. 208—9.

21. ibid., p. 193.

22. ibid., p. 198.

23. Inch, Sally, *Birthrights: A Parents' Guide to Modern Childbirth*, 2nd edition, London: Green Print, 1989, p. 90.

24. Dickersin, Kay, 'Pharmacological Control of Pain During Labour' in Chalmers et al., op. cit., 1989, p. 917.

25. Inch, op. cit., p. 115.

26. Haire, Doris, 'Drugs in Labor and Birth' in *Childbirth Educator*, Spring, 1987, pp. 1—7.

27. Clement, Sarah, 'Caesarean Childbirth: What are its Psychological Effects?', unpublished paper, 1990.

28. Moller-Pedersen, Kirsten, Thune-Larsen, Kari-Brith & Torgersen, Svenn, 'Psychologist at a Maternal Ward: Experiences and Evaluation of a Prevention Project' in *Nordisk Psykologi*, vol. 36, 1984, pp. 1—14.

Glossary of Terms

Accelerated labour When labour is speeded up artificially, by means of an intravenous drip administering a drug such as oxytocin.

Active birth A labour and delivery in which the woman follows her own instincts, is mobile and adopts upright positions such as kneeling, standing or squatting.

Active management of labour A policy of artificially rupturing the membranes early in labour, then using oxytocin to accelerate labour if the cervix is dilating at a rate of less than 1 cm per hour.

Amniotic fluid The liquid that surrounds the baby while he is in the uterus.

Anaesthesia Medication that takes away the sensation of pain.

Anaesthetic awareness When a general anaesthetic fails to render the patient fully unconscious, leaving her able to feel pain.

Analgesia Painkilling medication.

Antepartum haemorrhage Bleeding from the vagina in the last twelve weeks of pregnancy.

Anterior lip When dilation of the cervix is incomplete and part of the cervix is holding back the baby's head, the rest of the cervix being fully dilated.

Anterior position When the baby in the uterus lies in a head-down position with her back lying against the mother's abdominal wall.

Artificial rupture of membranes When a midwife or doctor breaks the bag of waters that surrounds the baby while he is in the uterus.

Aspiration A rare complication of general anaesthesia when the patient vomits while anaesthetised and the gastric contents are inhaled and enter the lungs.

Assisted vaginal delivery A birth in which forceps or a ventouse vacuum extractor are used to pull the baby out of the vagina.

Baby blues *See* Maternity blues.

Bikini cut *See* Lower segment incision.

Breech presentation When the baby is lying in a bottom-down rather than a head-down position in the uterus.

Brow presentation A position in which it is the baby's forehead rather than the crown of her head that is coming through the cervix first.

Caesarean section An operation where a baby is delivered through a cut in the mother's abdominal and uterine walls.

Catheter A fine plastic or rubber tube that is inserted into the bladder to empty it. *See also* Intrauterine catheter; Venflon catheter.

Cephalopelvic disproportion *See* Disproportion.

Cervix The entrance or neck of the uterus.

Classical incision A vertical cut running from the top of the uterus downwards, which is used in a minority of caesarean deliveries.

Clinical pelvimetry A vaginal examination carried out to give some indication of the size and shape of a woman's pelvis.

Continuous electronic monitoring Where the baby's heart rate is monitored continuously, via a monitor attached to a belt around the mother's abdomen (external monitoring) or via an electrode clipped onto the baby's scalp (internal monitoring). The monitors are attached to a machine that prints out a trace or graph of the baby's heart rate.

CPD *See* Disproportion.

Deep transverse arrest When the baby's head enters the mother's pelvis in a transverse (sideways) position and becomes stuck.

Dehiscence A small, benign and symptomless separation of a previous caesarean scar during a subsequent pregnancy or labour.

Disproportion When the baby will not fit through the mother's pelvis.

Distress *See* Fetal distress.

Drain A fine plastic tube that is sometimes put into a caesarean wound at the time of the operation to drain away any blood that might collect there.

Drip *See* Intravenous drip.

Dura A sheath of membrane that protects the spinal cord.

Dystocia *See* Failure to progress.

Elective caesarean A caesarean that is planned in advance.

Electrode A small electrical device which can be used to record a baby's or mother's heart rate.

Electronic fetal monitoring *See* Continuous electronic monitoring.

Emergency caesarean A caesarean that is not planned in advance, and is carried out when events during or before labour indicate that a caesarean is needed without much delay.

Engaged A baby is said to be engaged when his head (or bottom if it is breech) descends into the mother's pelvis, often in the last few weeks of pregnancy.

Epidural anaesthetic Regional anaesthesia, which is injected into the mother's spine (just outside the dura), to numb the lower part of the body, allowing a caesarean to be performed while the mother remains conscious.

Episiotomy A cut to the perineum to enlarge the vagina.

External monitoring Monitoring of the baby's heart rate either continuously via a monitor on a belt strapped around the mother's abdomen or intermittently using sonicaid or a fetal stethoscope.

External version When an obstetrician manipulates the mother's abdomen during the last weeks of pregnancy in an attempt to turn a breech baby from a bottom-down to a head-down position.

Face presentation When it is the baby's face rather then the crown of her head that is coming through the cervix first.

Failure to progress When labour is progressing slowly or stops. In the failure to progress during the first stage the cervix does not dilate at the required rate or stops dilating. In failure to progress during the second stage the baby does not descend into the vagina, or his descent is very slow.

Fetal distress A shortage in the flow of oxygen to the baby in her mother's uterus.

Fetal scalp blood sample When a small sample of blood is taken from the baby's scalp and analysed for its acidity and oxygen content, to indicate whether or not the baby is suffering from fetal distress.

Fetal stethoscope A stethoscope that is placed on the mother's abdomen to listen to the baby's heart.

Fetopelvic disproportion *See* Disproportion.

First stage of labour The phase of labour when the cervix is opening up until it is fully dilated.

General anaesthesia Anaesthesia that renders the patient unconscious and unable to feel pain.

Induction When labour is started off artificially by artificial rupture of membranes, the use of a vaginal pessary to prepare and soften the cervix and/or the use of an intravenous drip containing a drug such as oxytocin.

Intermittent fetal monitoring When the baby's heart rate is checked at regular intervals using either sonicaid or a fetal stethoscope.

Internal monitoring Monitoring of the baby's heart rate by means of an electrode attached to the baby's scalp.

Interuterine growth retardation When a baby in the uterus is not growing well and is smaller than would have been expected at a particular stage in pregnancy.

Intrauterine catheter A device inserted into the uterus during labour to measure the strength of contractions.

Intravenous drip A fine, hollow needle inserted into a vein in the hand and secured there with sticky tape. Fluids are passed into the bloodstream down a long tube and through the needle.

Inverted T incision A cut in the uterus which is shaped like an upside-down letter *T*. This cut is occasionally used during caesarean operations when it is difficult to get the baby out through a lower segment incision.

Intubation The passing of a tube down the trachea (windpipe) when general anaesthesia is being used.

IV *See* Intravenous drip.

Ketosis A condition in which lactic acid accumulates in a labouring woman's body tissues and fluids, altering the chemistry of her blood and weakening the muscle cells.

Late decelerations A sign of fetal distress, when the baby's heart rate takes a long time to return to normal after each contraction.

Lochia Bleeding from the vagina after childbirth, similar to a period.

Low lying placenta *See* Placenta praevia.

Lower segment incision A horizontal cut across the lower part of the uterus that is used in the majority of caesarean deliveries.

Malposition When a baby is lying in a head–down position, but his head is not in the ideal position for a vaginal delivery.

Malpresentation When some part of the baby other than her head, such as her bottom or shoulder, is the part that is coming through the cervix first.

Manual exploration of the uterus When a doctor inserts a hand into the uterus after a vaginal delivery to check the condition of a caesarean scar.

Maternity blues A period of tearfulness that typically occurs around four or five days after childbirth.

Meconium The first contents of a baby's bowel. If a baby passes meconium while still in the uterus this may be a sign of fetal distress.

Membranes The bag that holds in the amniotic fluid.

Mendelson's syndrome *See* Aspiration.

Midline incision *See* Classical incision.

Multiple pregnancy When there are two or more babies in the uterus.

Occipito posterior position *See* Posterior position.

Omnopon A morphine-based painkiller that is sometimes given after a caesarean birth.

Oxytocin A hormone that stimulates uterine contractions.

Para-median incision *See* Classical incision.

Partial shave Where the upper section of a woman's pubic hair is shaved off prior to a caesarean delivery.

Pelvic x-ray An x-ray of the pelvis carried out to determine the size and shape of a woman's pelvis.

Pelvimetry *See* Pelvic x-ray; Clinical pelvimetry.

Perineum The area between the vagina and anus.

Pethidine A morphine-based painkiller sometimes used during labour and after a caesarean birth.

Pfannensteil incision *See* Lower segment incision.

PH balance A measure indicating the balance of acid and alkaline in a sample of blood from a baby's scalp.

Placenta The afterbirth, the organ that develops on the inner wall of the uterus, through which the baby is nourished and receives oxygen.

Placenta praevia A condition in which the placenta is lying over the cervix, blocking the baby's exit.

Placental abruption A condition in which part of the placenta peels away from the wall of the uterus.

Posterior position When the baby is lying in a head-down position with his back against his mother's back, his face and limbs facing her abdomen.

Postnatal depression Any form of prolonged depression which occurs in the first year after childbirth.

Post-traumatic stress A psychological reaction to extreme stress including symptoms such as flashbacks, nightmares, insomnia and anxiety.

Pre-eclampsia A condition that affects a minority of pregnant women. It is characterised by high blood pressure, protein in the urine and water retention and can have serious effects on mother and baby if untreated.

Prolapsed cord When the baby's umbilical cord slips through the cervix into the vagina before the baby is born.

Prolonged labour *See* Failure to progress.

Regional anaesthesia Anaesthesia, such as epidural or spinal anaesthesia, which takes away pain sensations from part of the body, with the patient remaining conscious.

Respiratory distress A condition in which a baby suffers breathing difficulties after delivery.

Scan *See* Ultrasound scan.

Scar separation When the scar from a previous caesarean comes apart during a subsequent pregnancy or labour.

Second stage of labour The phase of labour during which the mother pushes the baby out.

Section *See* Caesarean section.

Shoulder presentation *See* Transverse lie.

Small-for-dates *See* Interuterine growth retardation.

Sonicaid A hand-held ultrasound monitor that is placed against the mother's abdomen to listen to the baby's heart rate.

Spinal anaesthetic Regional anaesthesia, which is injected into the mother's spine (into the cerebrospinal fluid at the centre of the spinal column), to numb the lower part of the body, allowing a caesarean to be performed while the mother remains conscious.

Spinal headache A very severe headache that can arise as a complication of spinal or epidural anaesthesia.

Spontaneous onset of labour When labour begins of its own accord.

Supplementary bottles Bottles of formula milk given to breastfed babies in addition to breastmilk.

Tracheal tube A tube that is passed down the trachea (windpipe) when general anaesthesia is used.

Transverse incision *See* Lower segment incision.

Transverse lie When a baby in the uterus is lying in a horizontal position across her mother's abdomen.

Trial of labour A situation in which there is some uncertainty about whether a vaginal delivery will be possible. The labour is watched carefully and everything is ready should the need for a caesarean arise.

Trial of scar The technical term for a trial of labour in a woman who has previously given birth by caesarean.

Ultrasound scan A way of visualising the baby inside the uterus by means of ultrasonic waves. A transducer is passed over the mother's abdomen and a picture of the baby appears on a screen.

Uterine rupture *See* Scar separation.

Uterus Womb.

VBAC A vaginal birth after a caesarean.

Venflon catheter A small hollow needle that is inserted in the hand to enable an intravenous drip to be inserted very quickly.

Ventouse vacuum extractor An instrument, used as an alternative to forceps, to help to pull the baby out of the vagina, by means of a suction cup which attaches to the baby's head.

Window Small areas of the lower body that remain unaffected by epidural anaesthesia. The term 'window' is also used to refer to a small benign scar separation or dehiscence.

Wound infection When the area where the caesarean incision was made becomes infected.

X-ray pelvimetry *See* Pelvic x-ray.

Further Reading

CAESAREAN CHILDBIRTH

Brooks, Melissa, *Caesarean Birth: A Guide for Parents*, London, Optima, 1989.

Duffet-Smith, Trisha, *You and Your Caesarean Birth*, London, Sheldon Press, 1985.

Francome, Colin, *Changing Childbirth: Interventions in Labour in England and Wales*, London, Maternity Alliance, 1989.

Maternity Alliance, *One Birth in Nine*, London, Maternity Alliance, 1986.

Philipp, Elliot, *Caesareans: An Explanation and Preparation*, London, Sidgwick & Jackson, 1988.

Reader, Fran & Savage, Wendy, *Coping with Caesareans and Other Difficult Births*, London, MacDonald, 1983.

VAGINAL BIRTH AFTER CAESAREAN

Cohen, Nancy Wainer & Estner, Lois J., *Silent Knife: Cesarean Prevention and Vaginal Birth after Cesarean*, Mass, USA, Bergin & Garvey, 1983.

Richards, Lynn Baptisti, *The Vaginal Birth after Cesarean Experience: Birth Stories by Parents and Professionals*, Mass, USA, Bergin & Garvey, 1987.

THE PSYCHOLOGICAL EXPERIENCE OF CHILDBIRTH

Ashford, Janet Isaacs, *Birth Stories: The Experience Remembered*, San Francisco, The Crossing Press, 1984.

Kitzinger, Sheila, *Giving Birth: How It Really Feels*, London, Gollancz, 1987.

MacFarlane, Aiden, *The Psychology of Childbirth*, London, Fontana, 1977.

Oakley, Ann, *Women Confined: Towards a Sociology of Childbirth*, Oxford, Martin Robertson, 1980.

Panuthos, Claudia & Bierkoe-Peer, Barbara, *The Emotional Ups and Downs of Childbirth*, Boston, People Place, 1981.

Price, Jane, *Motherhood: What It Does to Your Mind*, London, Pandora, 1988.

Raphael-Leff, Joan, *Psychological Processes of Childbearing*, London, Chapman & Hall, 1991.

PREGNANCY AND BIRTH

Balaskas, Janet, *New Active Birth: A Concise Guide to Natural Childbirth*, London, Thorsons, 1989.

Balaskas, Janet & Gordon, Yehudi, *The Encyclopaedia of Pregnancy and Birth*, London, MacDonald, 1987.

Enkin, Murray, Keirse, Marc J.N.C. & Chalmers, Iain, *A Guide to Effective Care in Pregnancy and Childbirth*, Oxford, Oxford University Press, 1989.

Inch, Sally, *Birthrights: A Parents' Guide to Modern Childbirth*, second edition, London, Green Print, 1989.

Kitzinger, Sheila, *New Pregnancy and Childbirth*, London, Michael Joseph, 1989.

Phillips, Angela, *Your Body, Your Baby, Your Life*, second edition, London, Pandora, 1991.

BREASTFEEDING

Kitzinger, Sheila, *Breastfeeding Your Baby*, London, Dorling Kindersley, 1989.

Messenger, Maire, *The Breastfeeding Book*, London, Century, 1982.

National Childbirth Trust, *Breastfeeding After a Caesarean Section*, leaflet, London, NCT, 1990.

POSTNATAL DEPRESSION

Comport, Maggie, *Surviving Motherhood*, Bath, Ashgrove Press, 1989.

National Childbirth Trust, *Mothers Talking about Postnatal Depression*, leaflet, London, NCT, 1983.

Welburn, Vivienne, *Postnatal Depression*, London, Fontana, 1986.

LOSING A BABY

Borg, Susan & Lasker, Judith, *When Pregnancy Fails: Coping with Miscarriage, Stillbirth and Infant Death*, London, Routledge & Kegan Paul, 1983.

Kohner, Nancy & Henley, Alix, *When a Baby Dies*, London, Pandora, 1991.

RIGHTS AND ASSERTIVENESS IN CHILDBIRTH

Beech, Beverley Lawrence, *Who's Having Your Baby? A Health Rights Handbook for Maternity Care*, London, Camden Press, 1987.

Dickson, Anne, *A Woman in Your Own Right*, London, Quartet, 1982.

Kitzinger, Sheila, *Freedom and Choice in Childbirth*, Harmondsworth, Penguin, 1988.

Wesson, Nicky, *The Assertive Pregnancy*, London, Thorsons, 1988.

Useful Addresses

Please send a s.a.e. when writing to these organisations.

Active Birth Centre, 55 Dartmouth Park Road, London NW5 1SL (071 267 3006). Antenatal classes, yoga for pregnancy and counselling.

AIMS (Association for Improvements in the Maternity Services), 40 Kingswood Avenue, London NW6 6SL (071 278 5628). Support and information about arranging the kind of birth you want, making a complaint and other aspects of maternity care.

Association for Postnatal Illness, 25 Jerdan Place, London SW6 1BE (071 386 0868). Support and information for those suffering from postnatal depression.

Association of Breastfeeding Mothers, Sydenham Green Health Centre, Holmshaw Close, London SE26 4TH (081 778 4769). Support and information on breastfeeding.

Birth Crisis Network, phone Sheila Kitzinger on 0865 300266 for the number of your nearest counsellor. Woman-to-woman telephone support for anyone who has had a bad or difficult birth experience.

Blisslink, 17 – 21 Emerald Street, London WC1N 3QL (071 831 9393). Support for parents of babies who are (or have been) in special care.

Boulton Hawker Films, Hadleigh, Near Ipswich, Suffolk IP7 5BG (0473 822235). Distributes (for hire or purchase) a video entitled 'A Baby by Cesarean'.

British Association for Counselling, 37a Sheep Street, Rugby CV21 3BX (0788 578328). Provides a list of qualified counsellors and psychotherapists in your area.

British Association of Psychotherapists, 121 Hendon Lane, London N3 3PR (081 346 1747). Provides a list of qualified psychotherapists in your area.

Caesarean Support Network, c/o Sheila Tunstall, 2 Hurst Park Drive, Huyton, Liverpool L36 1TF. Information and support for those facing a caesarean, those who have had a caesarean and women who are seeking a vaginal birth after a previous caesarean. Has a network of support groups throughout Britain. Information on obtaining videos about caesarean birth.

Community Health Council, address and phone number in local telephone directory. Offers information on local health services, and on obtaining the type of health and maternity care you require. Also offers advice and support to those who wish to make a complaint.

Independent Midwives Association, 74 Aukland Road, London SE19 2DH. Provides a list of independent midwives who offer private maternity care for home (and sometimes hospital) births.

La Leche League, Box 3424, London WC1N 3XX (071 404 5011). Support and information on breastfeeding.

National Childbirth Trust, Alexandra House, Oldham Terrace, London W3 6NH (081 992 8637). Offers antenatal classes, postnatal and breastfeeding support. Publishes leaflets on 'Caesarean Birth' and 'Breastfeeding after a Caesarean Section'. Runs a network of caesarean support groups around the country.

Relate (formerly the Marriage Guidance Council), address and phone number of local branch in local telephone directory. Offers counselling to individuals and couples experiencing difficulties in relationships.

SANDS (Stillbirth and Neonatal Death Society), 28 Portland Place, London W1N 4DE (071 436 5881). Offers support to parents whose babies are born dead or die soon after birth.

Society to Support Home Confinement, Lydgate, Lydgate Lane, Wolsingham, Bishop Auckland, County Durham DL13 3HA (0388 528044). Support for those seeking a home birth.

V.B.A.C. Information and Support, c/o Linda Howes, 8 Wren Way, Farnborough, Hampshire GU14 8SZ (0252 543250). Support and information for those seeking a vaginal birth after a caesarean.

Wide Awake Club, c/o Rita Sharples, 8 St Anne's Court, Shevington, Nr Wigan WN6 8HL. Support for those who have experienced pain during an operation under general anaesthetic.

AUSTRALIA

International Childbirth Education Association, National Co-ordinator Julia Sundin, 14 Clermisdon Avenue, Roseville, NSW 2069.

Parents' Centres Australia, 45 Albion Street, Harris Park, NSW 2150.

NEW ZEALAND

International Childbirth Education Association, National Co-ordinator Jenny Drew, 102 Cannington Road, Dunedin, Otago 9001.

Federation of New Zealand Parent Centre Incorporated, PO Box 17 — 351, Wellington.

Index

acceleration of labour *see* oxytocin drip

acceptance, of caesarean *see* coming to terms

active birth, 196

active management of labour, 36-7

afterpains, 79

anaesthesia: acupuncture, 56; choice of, 52-6, 57; hypnosis, 56; *see also* epidural anaesthesia; general anaesthesia; spinal anaesthesia

anaesthetic failure, 56, 65-7

anger, feelings of, 43, 93-6, 106, 110, 117, 145

antenatal classes, 44-5, 201, 205

antepartum haemorrhage, 28-9

anterior lip, 20

anterior position, of baby, 25-6

artificial rupture of membranes, 22, 37, 181, 199

aspiration, risk of, 58, 183-4

assertiveness, 177, 187

baby blues, 83-4, 108

Balaskas, Janet, 197

bathing, after caesarean, 77

Beech, Beverley Lawrence, 159

betrayal, feelings of, 105-7

Bettleheim, Bruno, 131

birth attendants, 198

birth plan, 70

blood transfusion, 89-90

body, feelings about, 102, 119, 123

bonding, 111-14, 119, 123, 142-3; *see also* mother-child relationship

bottle feeding, 122-3, 124

bowel movements, after caesarean, 77

breastfeeding, 115, 118-24, 204

breech baby, 23-5, 33, 68, 197; exercises to turn, 197; VBAC, 176

brow presentation, 25, 26

caesarean birth: attitudes towards, 40-8; description of operation, 58-60; feelings after, 13-15, 84-5, 91-2, 91-110; feelings during, 60-5

caesarean birth alternatives, 190, 202-4

caesarean birth rates, 17, 32-9, 182, 196, 206-7

caesarean-born children: explaining caesarean to, 129-32, 153; feelings of, 127-32; mother's perceptions of, 124-7

caesarean prevention, 195-201

caesarean support groups, 154, 177, 201, 202

Caesarean Support Network, 15, 134, 136, 138, 181, 182

caesareans: first, 109, 113; gap between, 164; number of, 17, 59, 166; subsequent, 164-71, 188-92

care *see* support

caring for baby, 80-2

catheter, 57, 75-6

cephalopelvic disproportion (CPD) *see* disproportion

classical incision, 26-7, 59, 120, 172-3, 179

Cohen, Nancy and Estner, Lois, 97, 130, 153, 165, 182, 185, 193

coming home, 84-8, 117

coming to terms, with caesarean, 44, 131, 149-63, 193-4, 210

complaint, making a, 158-9

complications, of caesarean, 14, 47, 89-91, 99, 135

consultant *see* obstetrician

convenience, as reason
  for caesarean, 36, 69
cord, umbilical, 22, 24;
  see also prolapsed
  cord
court-ordered
  caesareans, 71

death of baby, 31,
  117-18
deep transverse arrest,
  26
defensive medicine, 35
denial, feelings of, 91-2
diabetes, 31
dilation of cervix, 18,
  19, 20, 37
disproportion, 18-19,
  20, 23, 102, 173-5,
  197
distress *see* fatal distress
domino delivery, 181,
  196
drain, 60, 75-6
drip *see* intravenous
  drip
driving, after caesarean,
  86
dystocia *see* failure to
  progress

elective caesarean, 19,
  50-1, 169-70, 189,
  203
emergency caesarean,
  49-50, 91, 94, 109,
  113, 124, 135
empowerment, 16, 70
engagement, of fetal
  head, 18-19
English, Jane
  Butterfield, 128-9
Enkin, Murray, and
  colleagues, 71, 175,
  178, 199
entonox, 67, 200
envy, feelings of,
  99-100
epidural anaesthesia, for
  caesarean: failure of,
  66-7; feelings
  relating to, 62-5,

189, 208; and
  presence of partner,
  137-40; pros and
  cons of, 52-6, 80,
  169; setting up, 57-8;
  and trial of labour,
  186
epidurals, during
  labour, 21, 22, 200-1
episiotomy, 23, 24, 41,
  160-1
exercise: after caesarean,
  87; during
  pregnancy, 196
exercises: to turn
  breech baby, 197; to
  turn posterior baby,
  197
expectations: about
  caesarean birth, 16,
  40, 67, 157-8, 159;
  about vaginal birth,
  14, 40-3, 67, 70, 96,
  99, 144
explanations, 43, 69,
  87-8, 91, 115, 145,
  157, 206-7
external version, 24-5,
  197

face presentation, 25,
  26
failure, feelings of,
  100-1, 117, 119, 125,
  144, 165, 170
failure to progress,
  19-21, 100, 174-5
father *see* partner
father-child
  relationship, 142-3
female identity, feelings
  about, 101-2, 119
fetal distress, 18, 20,
  21-3, 35, 143, 181,
  198-200
fetal heart monitoring
  see monitoring
fetal scalp blood
  sample, 22, 200
fibroids, 32
forceps, 21, 23, 24, 26,
  29, 32, 35, 160

general anaesthesia, for
  caesarean: failure of,
  65-6; feelings
  relating to, 60-2, 94,
  98-9, 103, 156, 189,
  206; and presence of
  partner, 134-7, 138,
  208; pros and cons
  of, 52-6; and
  relationship with
  child, 113, 125, 126;
  setting up, 58, 60
GP unit, 196
guilt, feelings of, 100,
  117, 141, 144, 151

health visitor, 85,
  154-5, 210
heart disease, 32
herpes, 31-2
home birth, 187-8, 196
home help, 86
hospital: changing, 138,
  177, 202; choosing a,
  196-7; when to go
  into, 180-1, 198, 203
hospital notes, 156-7
hospital stay, 74-84,
  204, 209; feelings
  during, 82-4, 91-2;
  length of, 84-5, 209
housework, after a
  caesarean, 86
Huntingford, Peter, 34,
  135, 136
hysterotomy, 173

identity, 100-2
incision, types of, 58,
  173; *see also* classical
  incision; scar
induction, of labour,
  20, 30, 101, 186,
  197-8
infection: in baby,
  19-20; after
  caesarean, 47, 87,
  185; *see also* wound
  infection
infertility, 31, 47
information, 16, 43, 44,
  67, 115, 201

informed consent, 43, 56, 70-1, 207
interuterine growth retardation, 30
intervention: cascade of, 54, 69, 198; levels in trial of labour, 28, 178, 180-7
intrauterine catheter, 182
intravenous drip (IV), 57, 75-6, 182-3
intubation, 58, 79, 135
involvement in decisions, 69-71, 94, 106, 113, 144-5, 192, 208

ketosis, 183-4
Kitzinger, Sheila, 70, 104, 113, 197; and Celia Kitzinger, 130
Klaus, Marshall and Kennel, John, 113-14

labour: experience of, 96-7, 169, 170; first stage of *see* dilation of cervix; length of, 19-21, 38, 198; second stage of, 20-1, 23, 185
lifting, after a caesarean, 86
lochia, 76
loss, feelings of, 15, 44, 96-100, 115, 118, 206

making love, after caesarean, 86-7, 105, 147, 160-1
male attitudes, 38-9
malposition, 20, 25-6, 29
malpresentation, 28, 29
manual exploration of the uterus, 185
maternal age, 20, 32, 33, 176-7
meconium, 21, 22, 199
midwives, 85, 154-5, 178, 188, 196, 210

missing information, 98, 155-8
missing out, feelings of, 99-100
mobility: after caesarean, 76, 86; during labour, 20, 37, 181, 183, 198
monitoring, of fetal heart, 21-2, 199-200; and caesarean rates, 35, 37-8, 182, 200; in trials of labour, 181-2
mother-child relationship, 111-32, 188
mortality: feelings about, 102-5; maternal, 47, 180; perinatal, 34, 180

necessity, perceptions of, 68-9, 94, 106, 145, 192, 207-8
nutrition: after a caesarean, 76-7; during pregnancy, 196; during trial of labour, 182-4

obstetrician: changing, 138, 171, 177, 202; choosing an, 196-7
obstetricians: attitudes of, 38-9, 47, 134-6; and caesarean rates, 36, 196
Odent, Michel, 24, 196
oxytocin drip, 20, 22, 37, 186, 199

pain: after caesarean, 41, 78-80; during caesarean *see* anaesthetic failure; of labour, 40-1; in scar, 86, 179, 186; during sex, 87
pain relief: after caesarean, 79-80, 204; during labour,

200-1
Panuthos, Claudia, 110; and Romeo, Catherine, 118-61
partner: feelings of, 133, 142, 143-6; present or not present at caesarean, 55, 133-42; relationship with, 146-8; supporting caesarean mother, 82, 147-8
passing urine, after caesarean, 77
pelvimetry, clinical, 174; x-ray, 18, 19, 23, 88, 177, 174
pelvis, size of, 18, 23, 102, 171, 173-5
pethidine: after caesarean, 80, 99; in labour, 200
placenta praevia, 28
placental abruption, 29
position, of mother in labour, 20, 22, 37, 183, 196, 188, 200
positive feelings: about baby, 111, 116, 125, 160; about caesarean, 93-5, 130, 148, 150-1, 160-1, 163, 165, 192; during caesarean, 15, 60-1; of partner, 137, 139-40, 141-2, 143, 145-6
post-traumatic stress, 107
posterior position, of baby, 25-6, 29, 197
postnatal depression, 43, 74, 99, 107-10, 125-6, 162, 165, 188
pre-eclampsia, 31
pregnancy, after a caesarean, 95, 151, 164-7
premature baby, 29, 30, 33, 48, 59
preparation, for

caesarean, 14, 44–5, 67, 190, 201, 205
previous caesarean: more than one, 27, 172; as reason for caesarean, 26–8, 68, 167–78
prolapsed cord, 29–30
prolonged labour *see* failure to progress

Raphael-Leff, Joan, 106, 116
reasons for caesarean: medical, 17–32; non-medical, 17, 35–9
recovery: emotional, 91–2, 149–63; physical, 16, 46, 88–91, 164, 190
respiratory distress, 48
risks: of caesarean, 46–8; of trial of labour or repeat caesarean, 26, 168, 180
rupture, of caesarean scar *see* scar separation

sadness, feelings of, 93–6, 98, 99, 110, 161–3, 191
Savage, Wendy, 34, 175
scan, ultrasound, 23, 28, 171
scar: appearance of, 88–9; feelings about, 105, 191; pain in, 88, 179, 186; *see also* incision; classical incision
scar separation, 26, 32, 47, 168, 172–3, 175, 176, 178–80, 182, 185

separation, after birth, 113–14, 116, 153, 208–9
shaving, of pubic hair, 56–7, 184
shock, feelings of, 49–50, 91–2, 117
shoulder presentation *see* transverse lie
six-week check, 87–8, 157, 207
size, of baby, 31, 174; *see also* disproportion
sleep, 75, 77–8, 81–2, 84
special care, babies in, 114–17, 208–9
spinal anaesthesia, 52–3, 57–8
spinal headache, 52, 90
squatting, during labour, 18, 196, 198
staff shortages, 36, 74, 210
sterilisation, 147, 166–7
stitches, 60, 76
support: for breastfeeding, 123–4; during caesarean, 139–40; at home, 85; during hospital stay, 74, 209; importance of, 42–3, 72–3, 94, 106–7, 109, 113, 145, 192, 207–8; during labour, 20, 72
surgery, feelings about, 102–3

talking, about caesarean, 151–5
TENS (transcutaneous electronic stimulation), 200
time limits: on labour, 19, 38; in trials of

labour, 28, 184–5
tiredness, 77–8, 87, 89
transverse lie, 25, 59
trial of labour: with breech, 24; for suspected disproportion, 19
trial of labour after previous caesarean (trial of scar), 26–8, 167, 178, 180–7; and epidurals, 186; and intravenous drip, 182–3; and monitoring, 181–2; nutrition during, 182–4; and oxytocin, 186; and time limits, 28, 184–5
triplets, 31, 59, 176
twins, 30–1, 120, 176

VBAC (vaginal birth after caesarean): breech, 176; feelings following, 165, 167–8, 193–4; rates, 168, 172, 173–4, 184; support group, 177; twins and triplets, 176; in USA, 167–8
ventouse, 21; *see also* forceps
video, of caesarean, 156, 190, 201, 203
violation, feelings of, 104–5

wind, after caesarean, 76, 79
wound infection, 47, 90–1, 176
writing, about caesarean, 152–3

x-ray, of pelvis *see* pelvimetry